A BE BETTER NOW BOOK

BE HAPPIER NOW

100 Simple Ways to Become INSTANTLY Happier

Written by **JACOB SAGER WEINSTEIN**

Illustrated by **LAUREN RADLEY**

NEW YORK

T0035817

For Teme and Jeff, with love

"Happiness is a how, not a what;
a talent, not an object."

—attributed to Hermann Hesse

An imprint of Macmillan Children's Publishing Group, LLC
120 Broadway, New York, NY 10271 • OddDot.com
Odd Dot ® is a registered trademark of Macmillan Publishing Group, LLC

Joyful Books for Curious Minds

Text copyright © 2023 by Jacob Sager Weinstein
All rights reserved.

The Be Better Now Series is a trademark of Odd Dot.

WRITER Jacob Sager Weinstein
ILLUSTRATOR Lauren Radley
DESIGNERS Tim Hall and Caitlyn Hunter
EDITOR Justin Krasner
VETTER Matthew D. Della Porta, PhD

Library of Congress Cataloging-in-Publication Data is available.

ISBN 978-1-250-79510-6

Our books are available at special discounts when purchased in bulk for premiums and
sales promotions as well as for fund-raising or educational use. Special editions or book
excerpts also can be created to specification. For details, contact the Macmillan Corporate
and Premium Sales Department at (800) 221-7945 ext. 5442, or send an email to
MacmillanSpecialMarkets@macmillan.com.

First edition, 2023
Printed in China by Hung Hing Printing

10 9 8 7 6 5 4 3 2 1

CONTENTS

HAPPY HEART 63

INTRODUCTION

It's easy to be happy. All you have to do is lose twenty pounds, double your salary, and buy that expensive car you've been dreaming about . . .

. . . except that the science is clear: Doing those things won't actually affect your long-term happiness. Studies have found that once the excitement of winning fades, lottery winners aren't much happier than they were before they hit the jackpot. And while exercise will, indeed, make you happier, you don't need to drop five sizes to reap its benefits. You just need to *move*.

In fact, as decades of research show, happiness isn't about what you have and what you look like. It's about how you think and what you do. And within this book, you'll find 100 simple things you can do right now.

Remember, though: That's 100 things you *can* do, not 100 things you must do. If you make any of them regular parts of your life, congratulations! Be sure to celebrate your success (page 70). But don't pressure yourself to change your life in 100 ways overnight. Set a compassionate goal (page 116) of making small changes. You'll be delighted at how they add up. I hope this book will make an immediate and positive difference in your life. Nothing could make me happier.

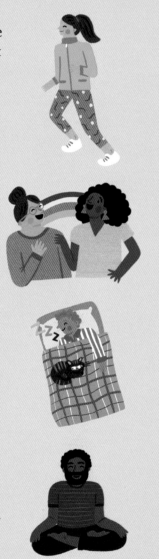

Correlation vs. Causation

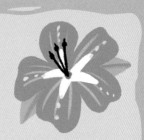

I've presented the science behind this book as simply and clearly as I can. But one concept is worth diving into more deeply: correlation vs. causation.

Correlation means that two things are likely to occur together. It's usually a two-way street. Being tall is correlated with being able to reach stuff on the highest shelf, and easily reaching high stuff is correlated with being tall.

Of course, some tall people can't reach high things because they have bad backs. Some masters of reaching high things are short people with ladders. Correlation doesn't mean that two things always go together—just that they tend to.

Causation means that one thing causes another. It often goes in one direction. Being tall causes you to reach high things more easily, but getting things off the top shelf doesn't make you taller.

Sometimes two things are correlated even though neither causes the other. Based on my extensive personal research, eating ice cream is correlated with getting a sunburn. Of course, neither one makes the other happen. The two things have a common cause—they're both caused by sunny weather.

Throughout this book, when I'm talking about correlation, I'll use phrases like "correlated with" or "associated with" or "linked to."

Read on—and be happier NOW.

ICONS TO LOOK FOR:

To help you zoom in on the tips that will make you the happiest, you'll find these icons throughout the book.

HABITS

Some things in this book are one-time lessons to learn. But others are habits you can implement, becoming a little happier each time. If you want help on establishing good habits, see page 132. And if you want a habit tracker, there are some built right into the inside jacket of this book.

In researching this book, I noticed four elements that kept popping up as crucial elements in a happy life. I call these the **Felicitous Four**. They are:

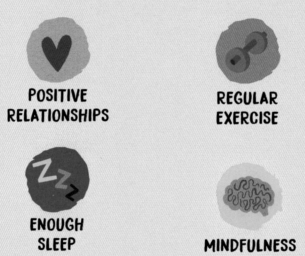

POSITIVE RELATIONSHIPS

REGULAR EXERCISE

ENOUGH SLEEP

MINDFULNESS

You're probably not surprised by any one of the Felicitous Four. But some of the details might surprise you—how little exercise you need to boost your mood (page 56), or when and how long a psychologically optimal nap is (page 49). Throughout this book, I've drilled down to the scientifically established specifics that change big, intimidating categories like "Mindfulness" into concrete things you can do *right now*.

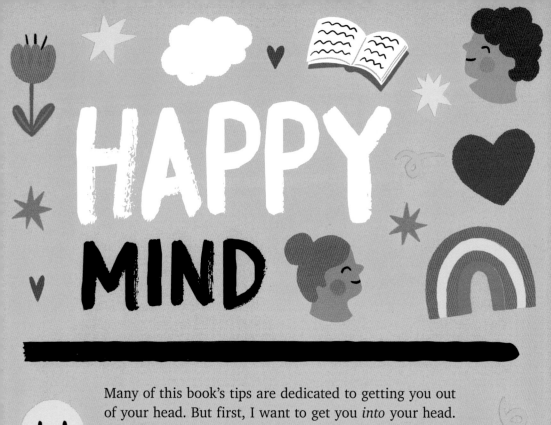

HAPPY
MIND

Many of this book's tips are dedicated to getting you out of your head. But first, I want to get you *into* your head. In this section, I'll offer mind tools to help you understand happiness, vocabulary to help you define it, and mental exercises to help you practice it.

THROW OUT THIS BOOK

Welcome to this book-length list of things you can do to be happier. Here's my first tip:

Don't make lists of things you can do to be happier.

In one small but suggestive study, scientists randomly assigned people to two groups. One was asked to write down ten things they could do to become happy. The other was asked to list ten things that showed they were *already* happy.

Afterward, the group that made a list of things to do felt less happy because they felt more strapped for time.

Obviously, I don't really want you to throw out this book. But the study brings up an excellent point: If you already feel you have too much on your plate, treating happiness as just another household chore can make

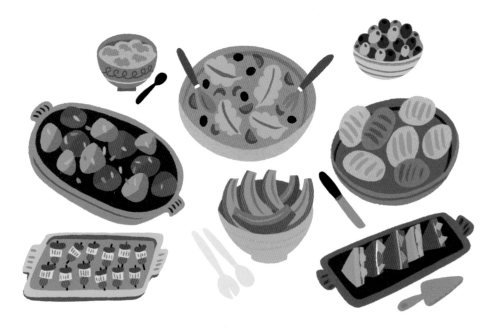

you miserable. Please don't view *Be Happier Now* as a lengthy to-do list! Instead, think of it as a happiness buffet. If you eventually sample every dish, that's wonderful. But if you just nibble a few random items—or if you don't try any of my dishes, instead using them as inspirations for your own recipes—that's great, too.

And before you start in on my buffet, why not take some time to appreciate the things you've already got in your pantry? (I'm hoping a love of painfully extended metaphors is one of them.)

STEP 1: Write down a few things you're already happy about. If you can't think of any, that's okay! Write down a few things you're grateful for, or you're looking forward to, or that went well recently. Or write down things you're already doing to improve your happiness. Buying this book counts! So does drinking coffee (page 41).

STEP 2: If you couldn't generate any answers in Step 1, that's okay, too. But you may want to look at page 134.

STEP 3: Realize there's no pressure to do any other exercise in this book.

☐ If you could do any part of Step 1, you're off to a great start.

THINK LIKE A PSYCHIATRIST

Throughout this book, I'll talk about different ways to define happiness. Understanding those definitions can help you understand your own emotions better—and that's a recipe for happiness, however you define it.

For now, let's look at how psychologists define it . . . and, for that matter, what psychologists are.

Psychologist vs. Psychiatrist vs. Psychotherapist

- A **psychologist** studies human behavior. They may have a PhD, but they don't have a medical degree. The research this book is based on was mostly done by psychologists.

- A **psychiatrist** is a medical doctor with a specialization in mental health.

- A **psychotherapist** works with patients to help them overcome mental health problems. A psychotherapist can be a psychologist, a psychiatrist, or another mental health professional . . . but it can't be a book. If you think you might benefit from therapy, see page 134.

How Do You Measure Happiness?

Throughout the book, I'll introduce many ways of measuring happiness. For starters, let's talk about *affective well-being* vs. *cognitive well-being*.

Affective well-being measures how you *feel* in this particular moment. If you're happy or hopeful, you have **positive affect.** If you're anxious or angry, you have **negative affect.**

Cognitive well-being measures what you *think* about how you feel. Psychologists frequently measure this by asking people to reflect on their overall happiness rather than how they feel right then.

As you'd expect, these two kinds of well-being often go together—but they don't always. When your baby starts shrieking on a crowded bus, you probably would have negative affect—but if you feel blessed to have a healthy child with strong lungs, your cognitive well-being could still be high.

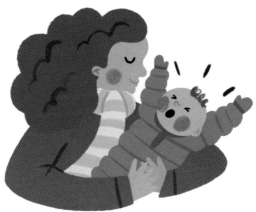

STEP 1: Understand the difference between affective well-being and cognitive well-being.

STEP 2: Think about how they apply to you. In this moment, is your affect positive or negative? Overall, do you feel happy with your life?

☐ If you better understand how mental health professionals think about happiness, you've won a greater understanding of yourself.

COPE APPROPRIATELY

When something's bothering you, there are many ways to cope. Some of them are inherently unhealthy, like drinking yourself into the hospital. Stick to the healthy ways, which include both **emotion-focused coping** and **problem-focused coping**.

Problem-focused coping deals directly with the thing that's bothering you. Emotion-focused coping deals with your reaction to it. If a witch has turned you into a frog, problem-focused coping might involve finding a prince or princess to kiss you. Emotion-focused coping might involve developing a taste for flies.

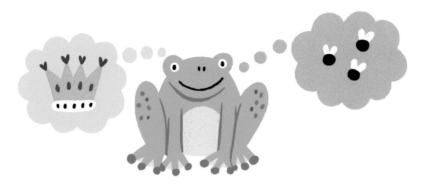

Neither kind of coping is inherently better than the other. In fact, they frequently work in concert with each other—often, you have to cope with your own emotions first, and once your head is on straight, you can start dealing with the problem itself.

In the sidebar, I've included some examples of both approaches. You'll notice that the emotion-focused coping methods are widely applicable, while any one problem-focused method is only useful in specific situations. That shouldn't be too surprising. There are a limited number of human emotions and an infinite number of circumstances that can trigger them.

Examples of Emotion-Focused Coping

Venting to a friend • Meditating • Exercising • Letting yourself cry it out

Examples of Problem-Focused Coping

Going to the doctor • Telling a friend how they hurt your feelings
Practicing to improve a skill • Hiring a plumber
Stealing the Declaration of Independence to read the treasure map on its back

STEP 1: Identify something that's troubling you.

STEP 2: Ask yourself: Is there something you can do to make it better in the short term? If so, go for problem-focused coping. Do what you can to make the situation better.

STEP 3: If there's nothing you can do right now or if you tried something and the problem still exists, switch to emotion-focused coping.

STEP 4: Once you're feeling a little better (or at least more in control), think about the long term. Is there any problem-focused coping you can do, even if it doesn't have an immediate payoff?

☐ If you've used one or both coping styles for one thing that's stressing you out, give yourself the win.

FIND YOUR FLOW STATE

Ever been so absorbed in a task that hours passed like minutes? And afterward, rather than being exhausted by the intensity, you were full of energy? If so, you've found **flow**. Besides healthy changes in your brain chemistry, flow states are correlated with a sense of purpose, orientation toward achievements, and happiness.

Mihaly Csikszentmihalyi coined the term "flow" in the 1970s and used this diagram to show that flow comes when your skills match the challenge you're facing.

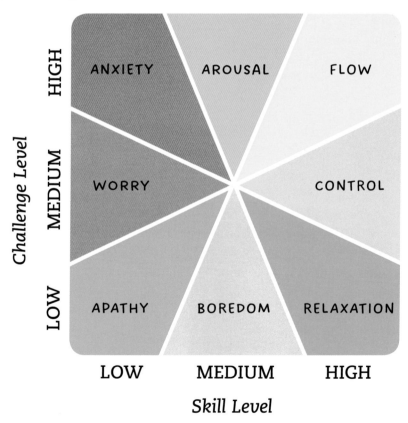

STEP 1: Take a risk. Danger activates focus, a key component of flow. You don't need to jump out of an airplane (although you could, if that's what gets your heart pumping). Giving a presentation to your colleagues counts, too. Whatever you do, it needs to require total concentration.

STEP 2: Take on a challenge. A close cousin to risks, challenges wake up our minds and senses, prompting our brains and bodies to fully engage with the task at hand. Make sure you have just enough skill to meet the challenge.

STEP 3: Make it new again. Fresh experiences can shake up your routine and wake up your mind, and new environments can engage all five of your senses and demand your full mind-body attention. Disrupt your established patterns just enough to engage your mind, but not so much that you find yourself flailing.

☐ If you lost track of time while making satisfying progress on an interesting task, flow straight into a victory.

CHECK YOUR GOAL ALIGNMENT

Numerous studies support the commonsense view that you're happier when you're moving toward your goals—but if your goals pull you in multiple directions, you'll always be moving away from one of them.

STEP 1: Write down your goals in life. List them by categories.

STEP 2: Is it logically possible to achieve all those goals at once? Does your goal of yarn-bombing a major monument on every continent conflict with your goal of always being at home with your family?

GOAL: Plan family-friendly yarn-bombing expeditions.

STEP 3: Think about the goals behind the goals. *Why* do you want to be with your family? Is it to share your passions with them? Use those *why*s to help craft new goals that are more in tune with one another.

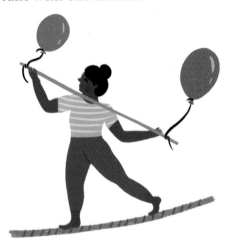

☐ If you've ferreted out and fixed at least one contradiction in your goals, make it your goal to accept the win.

What are my goals for my...

Job	Romantic life	Friendships	Family

Hobbies	Habits	Daily life	Everything else

LET GO OF UNHEALTHY SELF-GUIDES

The last exercise was about making sure your goals align with one another. But how do they align with *you*?

According to **self-discrepancy theory**, you're likely to be miserable when there's a big gap between your **self-guide** (your mental image of what you ought to be) and your **self-concept** (your mental picture of your messy, real-life self). You probably didn't need a fancy psychological theory to tell you that, but don't tell the psychologists. It might make them feel they're not living up to their ideal self-image as generators of surprising ideas.

The good news is that closing that gap can help us avoid unwanted negative emotions.

STEP 1: Think about a standard you feel you aren't meeting.

STEP 2: Reflect on where that standard came from. Is it one you truly believe in or something other people have imposed on you? Is it a realistic one for you to meet in the current circumstances of your life?

STEP 3: If it's a standard that you truly believe in, and one that you can realistically achieve, think about a realistic and self-compassionate plan for getting there. Otherwise, give yourself permission to drop it.

STEP 4: Take a quiet moment, and let yourself be aware of where you currently stand. Observe your messy desk as it is, not in comparison to the perfect desk that a better-organized you would have. If you feel judgments arise, observe them, too, and then let them go.

> ☐ If your self-concept (who you really are) feels even a tiny bit closer to your self-guide (who you believe you ought to be), be the kind of person who takes the win.

BE MORE YOU

On the last page, you let go of a standard that wasn't authentically you. Now it's time to replace it with one that is. You'll move a step closer to **authenticity**—the state of being true to yourself. That will cut down on **cognitive dissonance** (the difference between what you believe and what you do). And it will increase your **intrinsic motivation**—the drive that comes from pursuing meaningful goals.

STEP 1: Forget about the things you're supposed to want, and think about the things you really do want. Time with family? Creative satisfaction? Really good pizza? Focus on one that grabs you at this particular moment.

STEP 2: Think about a concrete step that frazzled, imperfect you can take to get closer to that goal. Imaginary Perfect You would organize the LEGOs by color and size, then work with your child to reconstruct the Taj Mahal. Actual You can dump the LEGOs on the floor and make glorified stick figures. Which you is going to have more real-life fun?

STEP 3: Go ahead and take that concrete step in your own imperfect way.

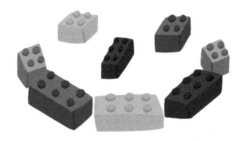

☐ If you gave yourself permission to do one thing that felt genuinely *you*, give yourself credit.

LEARN SOMETHING NEW

Learning has meaningful upshots for your happiness—not only can you fully engage your mind and trigger healthy changes in your brain chemistry, but your achievements can also spark joy and pride. Take some time to learn something new.

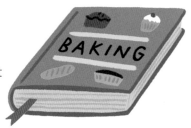

STEP 1: Find a new activity or skill (maybe something you've always wanted to learn) that's not too difficult or too easy. The right amount of challenge excites us, and the glee of overcoming it gives us the turbo-boost in happiness.

STEP 2: Take your first steps. Be easy on yourself when you judge the results. If it was something you could do right away, you wouldn't need to learn it. Bask in the satisfaction of starting off on a new path and celebrate any success you had.

STEP 3: Think about how you can expand your learning or skill even further next time—and how you can use your ever-improving skills to make the world a better place.

☐ If you've taken the first step toward learning a new skill, you're already learning how to make yourself happier.

KEEP LEARNING SOMETHING

The artwork for the last entry leaped from a cookbook to perfect cupcakes.

In reality, learning baking or any new skill can be frustrating and occasionally flour-covered. Research shows that people are more stressed and less happy when they're getting better at something. But those momentary lapses don't lessen their overall life satisfaction.

At heart, this gets back to the ancient Greek question of **eudaemonia** vs. **hedonia** (see page 102). Doing something you're bad at is never a source of pleasure, or hedonia. But sticking with it, and feeling the self-control that comes with growth and mastery, is a significant source of meaning, or eudaemonia.

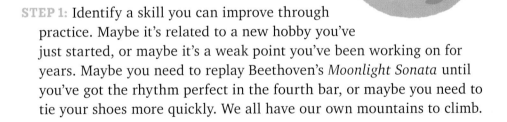

Or as more than one author has said: "I hate writing, but I love having written."

STEP 1: Identify a skill you can improve through practice. Maybe it's related to a new hobby you've just started, or maybe it's a weak point you've been working on for years. Maybe you need to replay Beethoven's *Moonlight Sonata* until you've got the rhythm perfect in the fourth bar, or maybe you need to tie your shoes more quickly. We all have our own mountains to climb.

STEP 2: No matter how badly you feel you're doing, keep practicing until you feel a sense of improvement. Trust that this effort will pay off over time, even if you don't feel very happy in the moment.

☐ If you've stuck with a skill you've already started to learn, give yourself a bonus win.

DECIDE!

Some say there are two kinds of people.
   (Let's make that pithier.)
There are two kinds of people.
   (Too definitive. Let's go back to the first version.)
Some say there are two kinds of people: **maximizers** and **satisficers**. Whether shopping for a car or writing a book, maximizers won't make a choice until they've found the absolute best option. Satisficers, by contrast, just want something good enough, and when they've found it, they'll accept it and move on. Maximizers might write more perfect sentences, but on average, satisficers feel . . . well, more satisfaction. They also feel less regret and jealousy.

STEP 1: Think about a decision you're facing.

STEP 2: List the concrete things that would make an option good enough.

STEP 3: Give yourself a deadline when the best good-enough option will become your final choice. Make it proportional to the significance of the choice. Choosing a new house? Give yourself a few months. Choosing where to order for dinner? That's ten minutes, max. (Tip: If you're a natural-born maximizer, maybe start with the dinner thing.)

STEP 4: When the deadline arrives, make the choice.

☐ If you've made a choice you can live with, choose to take the win.

SCHEDULE JOY . . . ROUGHLY

When you schedule something fun, you make it more likely to happen. You also make it feel more like work. The solution? Rough scheduling. Studies show that people enjoy roughly scheduled activities much more than formally scheduled ones.

STEP 1: Choose something you've been wanting to do.

STEP 2: Schedule it for a rough time frame. Think less "3:30 PM" and more "After I get home from work on Tuesday" or "The first sunny day this month."

STEP 3: Be equally rough in planning the end of your activity. A concrete deadline will hang over you the whole time, diminishing your enjoyment. "I'll hike until I start to get tired, then turn around" is great. "I better be back within fifty-nine minutes so I don't have to pay for a full hour of parking"? Not so great.

STEP 4: Don't schedule a second activity *after* your fun, even if it's an equally pleasurable one. If you can't dwell on your expectation of what's coming next, you're more likely to enjoy *now* as it happens.

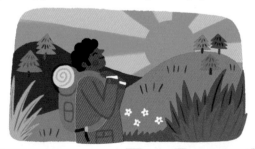

☐ If you've roughly scheduled one happy activity instead of planning it in detail, schedule taking the win for the moment you finish reading this sentence.

LOSE YOURSELF IN A BOOK

In the short term, reading has been found to diminish stress. In the long term, being swept away by literary fiction has been linked to improved empathy. Maybe that's not too surprising—any absorbing book will take you away from your own real-life problems, and a book focused on rich, nuanced characters can only help you understand your fellow human. "Hmmm," Jacob mused. "Can I transform this from a self-help manual into literary fiction, just by putting in dialogue?"

Try Finding a Book You Love...

- By an author who doesn't share your gender, sexual orientation, race, or religion.

- Translated from a language you don't speak.

- In a genre different from what you usually read.

- That's a graphic novel, audiobook, or other format you don't usually read.

- From a different era.

STEP 1: Find a book that will absorb you completely. If you love character-driven literary fiction, then by all means choose that to help build your understanding of the human condition. But the key is to choose something that will draw you in. Be guided by your own tastes rather than what you think you *should* want to read.

STEP 2: That said, reading a wide variety of books can help you to learn something new (page 14) and to find a link between yourself and different kinds of people (page 106). Consider looking for books you'll love in places you don't always look—see the sidebar for some suggestions.

STEP 3: However you've chosen your book . . . read it (or listen to it).

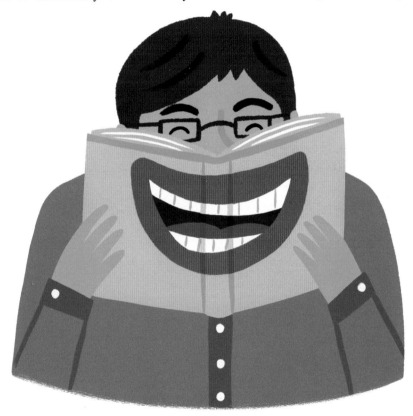

☐ If you spent six more minutes reading a book than you otherwise would have, shelve this one under "Victory."

ALL'S WELL THAT ENDS WELL

Your brain can't store everything you do. Instead, it takes snapshots, especially during peaks of intensity and at the end of an experience. Psychologists call this the **peak-end rule**. If a bad experience ends well, you leave with happier memories than if it simply ends.

Just ask any dentist who gives kids a toy as they're walking out the door. Even if you're not getting cavities filled, you can use the peak-end rule to make bad memories less bad and good memories even better.

STEP 1: Think about an upcoming event. Can you rearrange the order it occurs in so that it ends on the best bit (or the least worst bit)? Instead of meeting your obnoxious cousin at an ice-cream parlor and then heading to his place for an hour of excruciating conversation, swap it around so you can end on a hot fudge sundae.

STEP 2: If it doesn't have any good parts built in, can you add a pleasant note at the very end? If nothing can alleviate the misery of mowing the lawn, can you listen to your favorite song as soon as you go back inside?

☐ If you've ended one experience on a happier note than it otherwise would have, end by giving yourself the win.

STRENGTHEN HAPPY MEMORIES

You might not think of memory as a superpower, but it is. You can summon up and relive past events at will. How amazing is that? In the long run, even people who have had many miserable life events are less likely to suffer from depression if they can remember the happy ones.

As a bonus, every time you retrieve a memory, you make it less likely to fade. This is one superpower that gets stronger every time you use it.

STEP 1: Review a happy memory from the past twenty-four hours. Challenge yourself to recall it in as much detail as you can. It might help to describe the experience through your five senses—what did you see, smell, hear, taste, or touch?

STEP 2: Review a happy memory from about a week ago, and then from about a year ago. If you need to jog your memory, look at your calendar or your photo library. But it's the act of pulling a memory out of your own brain that helps you remember it, so ask yourself questions to go beyond the photo or calendar entry. What did you enjoy about that moment? Whom were you with? What led up to it, and what happened afterward?

STEP 3: During your daily life, keep an eye out for happy moments. Make a point of taking a mental recording that you can return to. (But don't do this at the expense of enjoying the moment as it happens!)

STEP 4: If you want to make life easier for Future You, consider starting a memory journal, with one memory-jogging note per day. I'm a little obsessive about this, so I use a flashcard app on my phone to actively quiz myself about my memories.

☐ If you've spent time reviewing happy memories (especially if it was a memory that you might have otherwise forgotten), remember to give yourself the win.

FOCUS ON THE NEGATIVE

Later in this book, I'll advise you to really focus on pleasurable experiences (page 55). But believe it or not, you'll be happier if you stay focused on not-so-great experiences, too.

That's because studies have shown that letting your mind wander during an unpleasant task is likely to make you less happy—even if your mind wanders to something pleasant. Maybe that's because fantasizing about a trip to Oahu while you're unclogging the toilet only emphasizes how smelly and dirty your immediate reality is.

Important caveat: We're talking garden-variety unpleasantness, like dealing with blocked plumbing. Anything that's truly horrible is beyond the scope of this book. Get through it however you can, then talk to a professional about it (page 134).

STEP 1: When you have to do something unpleasant, stay as present in the moment as you can. Don't wallow in your emotional reaction to it, but do stay aware of what your body is actually doing and how you feel about doing this task.

STEP 2: If you find yourself daydreaming, first notice that your mind has wandered. Then gently bring your attention back to the job at hand.

☐ If you've kept your focus on a negative task, focus on giving yourself the win.

BIAS YOURSELF

Was that clerk rude to you because you deserved it? Or were they just having a bad day? If you tend to pick the more upbeat choice, you have what's called a **positive interpretation bias**. It's the rare form of bias that can improve your life.

And fortunately, it's a form of bias you can acquire deliberately, through a technique that one study called "a cognitive vaccine." Like most vaccines, it's safe and effective. Unlike most vaccines, it'll leave you with a slightly more positive outlook instead of a slightly more swollen arm.

Note that you can do this exercise regularly to build up your positive interpretation bias, but you can also bust it out right before an anxiety-provoking event to help you approach it with a more positive attitude.

STEP 1: Think of a situation that could resolve positively or negatively—
for example, a party where you don't know anybody. Picture the setup
as vividly as you can, trying to engage all your senses, but once you've
got the image, don't linger on it too long. Move on quickly to . . .

STEP 2: Imagine a positive yet plausible resolution. Picture yourself
having a fascinating conversation with a stranger, who is so impressed
by your explanation of positive interpretation bias that they rush
right out and buy their own copy of *Be Happier Now*. (Well, that's my
visualization. Yours might be a little different.) Once again, imagine it
vividly, but don't linger on it too long.

STEP 3: Repeat the previous steps a couple of times.

☐ If you pictured one ambiguous event ending positively,
picture this exercise ending with a win.

EXPLAIN IT LIKE AN OPTIMIST

Pessimists do worse in school and at work. They're more likely to get sick and less likely to win elections. And they're more likely to suffer from depression.

To be clear, I'm talking about **pessimism** as defined by Martin Seligman, one of the pioneering researchers of the subject. Most of us would define pessimism as a belief about the future, but Seligman focuses mostly on how people explain the past.

In particular, Seligman says, when a pessimist explains a negative event, their explanation has three features:

- It's *personal*. It's the pessimist's own fault. "My dog escaped because I didn't spend enough money on a break-proof leash."

- It's *pervasive*. The problem extends well beyond this particular example. "I'm such an irresponsible pet owner. This is just like that time I accidentally stepped on Patch's paw."

- It's *permanent*. "I'll never deserve another pet."

By contrast, an optimist's explanation would have at least one of the following features:

- It's *impersonal*. It's not the optimist's fault. "Patch has such strong teeth, he would have chewed through any leash."

- It's *localized*. "Other than this, I've been a good pet owner. I groomed Patch regularly, I took him to the vet, and I even taught him how to drive a car."

- It's *temporary*. "Next time, I'll check the leash for wear and tear. Anyway, as soon as Patch runs out of gas, he'll call me."

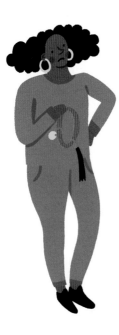

The good news is, pessimism itself is a temporary condition. Or at least it can be. With practice, you can learn to think like an optimist.

STEP 1: Think of something in your life that has a negative effect on your mood at the moment. It could be something big (like getting fired) or little (like the store being out of your favorite sliced bread).

STEP 2: Notice how you explain it. If your explanation is personal, pervasive, and permanent, challenge at least one of those aspects. Look for evidence that the problem is impersonal and/or localized and/or temporary.

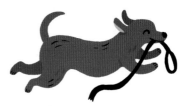

☐ If you've explained one thing the way an optimist would, explain to yourself that this was a win.

BLAST SOME ALIENS

When I was a kid, video games were a relatively new phenomenon. If I want to engage in nostalgia (page 81), all I have to do is listen to the original Pac-Man music, and I'm instantly transported back to my youth. Back then, there was something of a panic over this new art form, which was clearly going to transform children into violent, quarter-stealing game junkies.

Since then, psychological research has come to suggest the opposite: Under the right circumstances, video games can make you happier. Some games (like *Just Dance* or *Pokémon Go*) even combine the benefits of gaming with the benefits of exercise (page 56).

Maybe that's why moderate gamers are less likely to suffer from depression than nongamers.

Note the word *moderate*. Like any other pleasure, video gaming can become an addiction. As long as it's not out of control, video gaming can bring you joy. For maximum happiness, play video games . . .

- For fun. (And if you have to ask "What other reason would you play video games?", you've never felt the compulsion to complete 100 percent of a game's achievements long after you've stopped enjoying it.)

- With social aspects, especially cooperative ones (like joining with other players to achieve a quest). Even interacting with fictional characters may help.

- As part of a balanced social life that includes other forms of social interaction.

STEP 1: Find a video game you enjoy.

STEP 2: Play it for a fun but moderate period.

If you've played a video game today for a moderate period of time, you won at life.

IMAGINE THE GOOD, DESCRIBE THE BAD

Your thoughts affect your feelings—but some thoughts are more powerful than others. In particular, thinking in pictures has been shown to alter your mood more than thinking in words. Using words shifts brain activity away from the primitive emotion-processing circuitry of your amygdala, literally rerouting your thought process into more rational channels.

You can use that fact to make positive thoughts more vivid and negative thoughts more neutral.

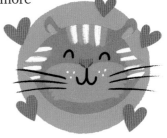

STEP 1: Think about something positive in your life—a person you love, say, or an event you're looking forward to. Imagine it in as much vivid, sensorial detail as you can.

STEP 2: Identify something that makes you anxious, like that root canal you've got next week. If images of it pop into your mind, don't judge them or fight them, but don't hang on to them, either. Imagine them floating away. Replace them with emotionally neutral words that describe how you're feeling.

I'm sweating and my heart is beating faster because I'm thinking about the dentist.

☐ If you've lingered on one happy image or replaced one negative one with neutral words, imagine getting a trophy.

TELL YOURSELF A STORY

One of the miracles of my profession is the way writing things down transforms my thoughts. Sometimes beliefs that seemed plausible inside my head are exposed as misunderstandings when I spell them out.

Other times the connection between two seemingly different ideas suddenly becomes clear, clicking them together in a newly coherent whole.

You don't have to be a writer to benefit. **Expressive writing**, as psychologists call the practice of putting your emotions on paper, has a host of well-demonstrated benefits. It can help prevent depression, improve relationships, and inspire self-doubters to believe in themselves. All it takes is fifteen minutes.

STEP 1: Think about a specific emotion or event that is bothering you. This could be something profoundly troubling, like a deep-seated fear, or superficially troubling, like a minor argument you had with a neighbor.

STEP 2: Set a timer for fifteen minutes. Use that time to write freely about the subject you've chosen. Don't worry about elegant prose or even correct spelling. Do make connections. What led to this event? Why did you feel the way you did? Have you experienced other events or feelings like this? What did they have in common, and how were they different?

STEP 3: When you're done, you can save your writing if you want to return to it—but you can also shred it. The important part was the process of writing it.

☐ If you've spent fifteen minutes putting your thoughts or feelings into words, take a second to think, "I did it."

GET IN A BORING ROUTINE

When you look ahead to something fun, you want to enjoy the anticipation (page 100). But the less you have to think about boring stuff, the better. Why let free-floating tasks loom over you? Assigning them specific times and places means you can forget about them for the other twenty-three hours and fifty-five minutes a day.

Plus, households with regular routines have been shown to better withstand crises. By establishing one now, you're providing yourself with a happiness insurance policy. When the zombie apocalypse comes, you'll find it surprisingly comforting to take the garbage out at the same time you always do. (Just make sure you put a zombie-proof lock on your trash cans. They're worse than raccoons.)

STEP 1: List the chores you have to do often. Which ones don't have specific rules about when they get done?

STEP 2: Come up with rules for when and where you'll do the free-floating chores. If there's more than one person in your household, considering assigning a "who" as well.

STEP 3: Stick to your routine until it becomes a habit.

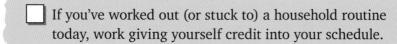

☐ If you've worked out (or stuck to) a household routine today, work giving yourself credit into your schedule.

RIDE THE MIND BUS TO HAPPINESS

Sometimes our thoughts are crammed with self-doubt, unhealthy impulses, and other things we'd rather be free of.

One promising technique for dealing with this is **cognitive defusion**. The idea is to separate who you are from what you are thinking in the moment. Instead of feeling fused to your thoughts and feelings, you *defuse* yourself from them.

If negative thoughts and feelings have a serious ongoing effect on your life, you should seek professional help (page 134). But for occasional negative episodes in which you feel tempted to do something you really don't want to do, a technique called the **mind bus** may help you drive forward into a happier life.

STEP 1: Picture your life as a bus and you as the driver.

STEP 2: Next time you feel negative impulses, think of them as passengers on the bus. They've bought their tickets, so they have a right to stay on the bus. But whether they're telling you to break your diet or yell at a loved one, *you* are the one at the steering wheel.

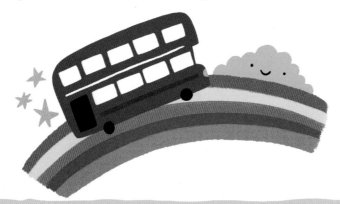

☐ If you've used the mind bus technique to resist a negative impulse, get off at the stop marked "Triumph."

DISPUTE NEGATIVE THOUGHTS

Sometimes disturbing thoughts refuse to sit at the back of the mind bus (page 30). In those cases, you can't ignore them. You need to dispute them. **Disputation** is a cognitive technique shown to help vanquish negative thoughts. If your negative thoughts are prosecuting you like attorneys in court, disputation lets you act as your own defense attorney.

Four elements will help your defense win the day:

Evidence. Often, negative thoughts run counter to the facts. Take a step back, and remind yourself of the evidence that things aren't as bad as they seem.

Alternatives. Even if your negative thoughts offer a plausible interpretation of the events, it can't be the only interpretation. Offer yourself alternatives.

Implications. Even if your negative thoughts have evidence on their side and even if they offer an accurate interpretation of the past, that doesn't mean they're correctly predicting the future.

Usefulness. Even a true statement isn't useful unless it moves you forward in life.

STEP 1: When you're confronted with negative thoughts, don't take them at their word. Dispute them.

I OBJECT!

STEP 2: Remember to use evidence, alternatives, implications, and usefulness to argue against the negative thoughts.

☐ If you've disputed one negative thought, feel positive.

IDENTIFY TIME VACUUMS

You have exactly 1,440 minutes per day. Sometimes you voluntarily spend them on things that make you happy. Other times they mysteriously disappear, leaving you frustrated and regretful.

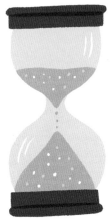

If sixty bucks were vanishing from your bank account every day, you'd investigate. Why would you put up with things that siphon away precious time? Fortunately, even small barriers can help us resist temptation.

STEP 1: Think about time that's gotten away from you recently. Did you sit down to spend five minutes on Twitter, only to lose twenty minutes? Turn on the TV to watch a half-hour sitcom, only to find yourself there two hours later? If you got joy and meaning out of the hours you spent, that's great! You can stop this exercise now. But if you regret the time, go on to . . .

STEP 2: Put barriers in place to delay you from starting this activity mindlessly. Delete Twitter from your phone, or put your remote control on a shelf you can't easily reach.

STEP 3: Next time you're about to start this activity, use the delay you created to think about the time it will *actually* cost you. What would you rather use that time for? Go do that, instead.

STEP 4: If you find it hard to resist temptation, tell yourself you're not giving up this mindless pleasure forever—just for now (page 114).

☐ If you've put a barrier between you and one time suck, vacuum up the win.

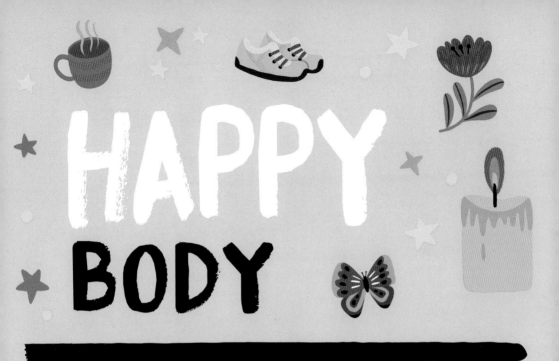

HAPPY
BODY

Sometimes happiness is a concrete thing. From savoring life's pleasures to getting a good night's sleep, this section will help you find happiness in the physical world.

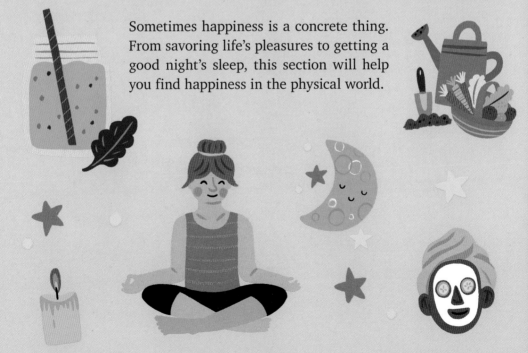

SAVOR THE GOOD STUFF

It's natural to think that your happiness depends on making good things happen. But it can be even more important to appreciate the good things you've already got. Researchers call this **savoring**. A study that tracked a random day in the life of **flourishers**—people with optimal mental health—found that they got more pleasure from simple daily experiences than nonflourishers. And the best news? Savoring is a skill that can be learned. You just have to take the time to do it.

I'm making this a separate tip because it's worth practicing on its own. But I hope you'll carry it over into pretty much every other suggestion I make. Savor everything that makes you happy!

STEP 1: Choose a simple pleasure. Don't make it a once-in-a lifetime luxury. You're looking for a pleasure you could enjoy on any random day.

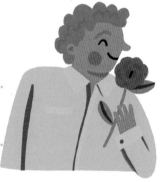

STEP 2: Give yourself enough time. You can't savor when you're rushing.

STEP 3: Pause distractions. Don't watch TV while you're eating that delicious apple. (For that matter—and I say this as a former TV writer—don't eat an apple while you're watching that perfectly crafted season finale.)

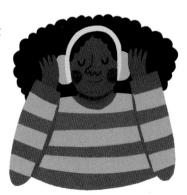

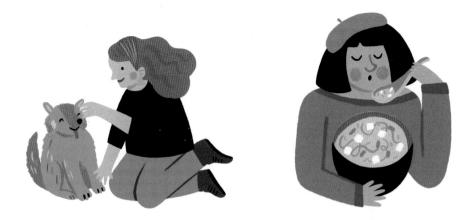

STEP 4: Your attention focused, dive in. Notice not just the big pleasures but also any subtleties along the way—the little hint of tartness that makes the apple's sweetness pop or the slight change in the protagonist's face right before the credits roll.

STEP 5: Enjoy the experience, and experience your own enjoyment.

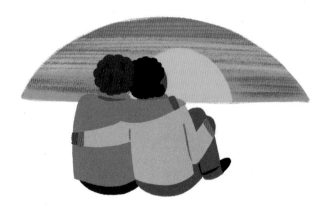

☐ If you've savored one delightful experience today, savor the win.

GET YOUR FINGERS DIRTY

Gardening combines fresh air, exercise, and exposure to nature. The result? It reduces your odds of depression and anxiety, and it increases your life satisfaction and sense of community, according to a meta-analysis of twenty-two studies that was definitely not done by rabbits posing as researchers. Rabbit-driven or not, the science is clear.

STEP 1: Find a suitable spot. Depending on where you live, that might be in your backyard or on a windowsill. It's also worth checking whether your neighborhood has a community garden, which would let you add social interaction to the list of benefits.

STEP 2: Get some soil and some seeds, and get digging. Or skip a step, and start with plants instead of seeds. Either way, if you're a beginner, start with something that's really easy to grow.

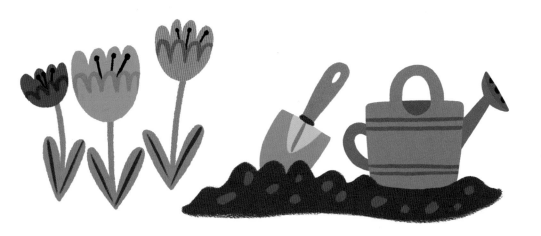

☐ If you've spent time today tending to a plant, you've planted the seeds of happiness.

WATER UP YOUR FEELINGS

In 2013, researchers checked in with twenty thousand smartphone users at random intervals to see how happy they were and where they were reporting from. People in any natural environment were happier than city dwellers—and people near the ocean were happiest of all. The effect remained even after scientists controlled for activity, so it wasn't just that beachgoers were more likely to be on vacation. Other studies suggest that even being near a fountain in a city environment can give you some of the same benefits as being by water in nature.

STEP 1: If you live near the coast, make a trip there.

STEP 2: If you don't live near the coast, plan a trip there.

STEP 3: If none of that is possible, get yourself to the nearest lake, river, or even public fountain.

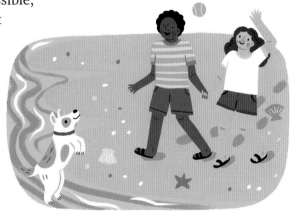

☐ If you've spent time today near a body of water (natural or man-made), you're swimming toward happiness.

CONNECT WITH NATURE WHEREVER YOU ARE

You might not have the space (or the inclination) to grow a garden (page 36). And even the hardiest happiness warrior can't get to a beach (page 37) or forest (page 39) every day. But connecting with nature is as much about your mental state as your physical location. A meta-analysis of twenty-one studies showed that people who merely *felt* connected to nature were more likely to be happy.

Psychologists haven't yet teased out cause and effect, but it's reasonable that simply feeling connected to all living things would have inherent psychological benefits.

STEP 1: Connect with nature in any way you can. Watch a documentary on a distant habitat, run your fingers on the leaves of the closest houseplant, or notice the grass growing in the cracks of the sidewalk.

STEP 2: Appreciate whatever bit of nature you're admiring, no matter how big or small it is. If you're watching a video, try pausing it on a particularly breathtaking frame. If it's in real life, take a photo of it (or draw a quick sketch if you'd prefer), thinking about how best to capture its beauty.

STEP 3: Think about what connects you to nature. Is it something physical, like breathing out carbon dioxide, which the plant needs to breathe? Is it something economic, like a donation you make to preserve that distant habitat? Or is it something intangible and spiritual?

☐ If you've made one connection with nature today, then give yourself credit, naturally.

TAKE A FOREST BATH

From *sushi* to *manga*, many Japanese words have made happy homes in the English language. It might be time to add *shinrin-yoku*, or "forest bathing," to the list. An array of biological and psychological studies show that *shinrin-yoku* slows pulses and reduces adrenaline, resulting in calmer moods and decreased rates of depression.

STEP 1: Find a wooded spot, whether that's Yosemite National Park, your backyard, or a local playground. If possible, don't take your phone or any other electronic devices. If you feel you need to take them, silence notifications and seal your devices in whatever container will help you avoid temptation.

STEP 2: Walk aimlessly and slowly. You're not trying to get anywhere in particular, which means there's no rush.

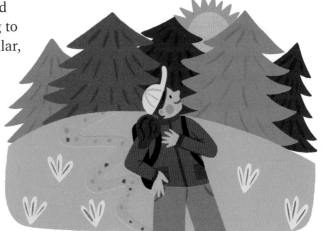

STEP 3: Engage with nature using all five senses. Listen quietly. Feel the texture of trees. But just use your sense of taste for sampling the fresh flavor of forest air. Unless you're an expert forager, I don't recommend licking random leaves.

☐ If you've forest bathed today (or backyard bathed, for that matter), you've grown some extra happiness.

FREE UP SPACE TO
FREE YOUR SPIRITS

When you feel your environment is cluttered, your levels of the stress hormone cortisol go up. I'm not talking about how somebody else might judge your environment. If those eight-foot-tall piles of newspapers are exactly what you want, then more power to you! Skip to the next page. (But don't literally skip. You might set off a newspaperlanche.)

For everybody else, even a small clean-out can give your body a little more room to move—and your spirit a little more space to breathe.

STEP 1: Set a timer for fifteen minutes.

STEP 2: Choose an area you'd particularly like to declutter, like a kitchen counter or a bedroom dresser. If you don't have a preference, look at the areas where you spend the most time and see what catches your eye as the most cluttered spot. Again, this is based on *your* feelings, not how you think anybody else might judge you.

STEP 3: Start tidying. When the timer dings, you're allowed to stop. (You're also allowed to keep going if you've got momentum.)

☐ If you've spent fifteen minutes decluttering, add an imaginary trophy to your shelf.

HAVE A CUPPA

When I moved to London twenty years ago, I finally understood why the British drink so much tea. It's the same reason Seattle is famous for coffee: On a dark, rainy day, nothing is more comforting than something warm and brightly caffeinated. It turns out that science agrees. In the short term, coffee and tea drinkers report more alertness and better moods. In the long run, they have lower risks of clinical depression.

Decaffeinated tea and coffee show some of the same benefits, but not all. Same for caffeinated water. That suggests there's something about the interaction between caffeine and the other components of tea and coffee that confers added benefits.

It's worth noting there is a limit. Too much caffeine can cause headaches, sleep disturbances, and potential other sources of misery. So have a drip brew—but not through an IV drip.

STEP 1: Brew a cup of coffee or tea.

STEP 2: Don't add sugar, which makes you more likely to crash later. If you can't stand the taste of unsweetened tea or coffee, try gradually reducing the amount of sweetener you add. Or dilute your brew by adding unsweetened creamer, dairy, or otherwise. Or just try a different variety—you might find you like a latte made with Ethiopian coffee beans more than a cold brew made with Salvadoran Bernardina.

STEP 3: Drink it. Try savoring the experience (page 34).

☐ If you've had a cup of tea or coffee today, drink in the victory.

BEAT THE WINTER BLUES

If, like me, you find yourself feeling genuinely miserable in winter, you may have SAD—seasonal affective disorder.

The problem? Lack of sunlight. Sunlight signals your brain to stop producing melatonin (which makes you sleepy) and start producing serotonin (which helps regulate your moods). Plus, your skin needs sunlight to produce vitamin D, which may also help keep your brain happy.

Fortunately, you can simulate the sun in your eyeballs with a SAD lamp. And you can simulate the sun on your skin with vitamin D pills. (Full disclosure: Studies on vitamin D have shown mixed results in treating depression. But they've shown unambiguous benefits for physical health and no drawbacks in the moderate dosages recommended below.)

A particular form of therapy called cognitive behavioral therapy has also been shown to help in treating SAD, but it's beyond the scope of this book. If the tips on this page don't have you feeling happier in a week or two, it's worth talking to a mental health professional (page 134). And if you're having thoughts of self-harm, don't wait even that long.

STEP 1: Get a SAD lamp. Look for one that offers something like 10,000 lux (a measurement of brightness) at the distance you'll be sitting from it. Make sure that it's from a reputable manufacturer (like Lumie or Philips) and that it has a UV filter to prevent damage to your eyes. Check the directions for your particular light to find out how long to use it each day.

STEP 2: Take a daily vitamin D supplement. The US RDA for most adults is fifteen micrograms or mcg (also known as six hundred international units or IU). When it comes to dietary supplements, more is *not* better. Doctors warn against taking more than one hundred mcg (four thousand IU) for grown-ups. Check with your pediatrician before giving any supplements to children.

STEP 3: Consider getting a sunrise alarm clock—a clock that wakes you up by gradually brightening your bedroom.

STEP 4: Plan a happy activity you associate with winter, like building a snowman or drinking hot chocolate. (See page 130 for more thoughts on celebrating the season.)

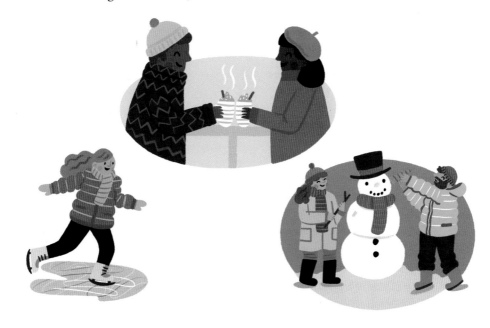

☐ If you've done one thing today to fight the winter blues, bundle yourself in triumph.

SLEEP ON IT

It's well-established—in science and probably in your daily life—that a good night's sleep predicts feelings of happiness. In fact, some studies suggest that getting enough sleep is the single biggest factor in feeling that you're living well.

Tips for Happy Sleep

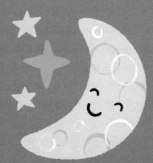

Keep cool. In the winter, set your thermostat for somewhere between sixty and sixty-seven degrees Fahrenheit. In the summer, rather than blast the air-conditioning, it might be cheaper to point a fan at your bed. However you do it, the right bedroom temperature can give you almost twenty minutes of extra sleep over the course of a night.

Program your internal clock by getting in and out of bed at roughly the same time every day. You might not believe it when you're dragging yourself out of bed, but in the long run, you'll be better rested.

Establish a consistent pre-bed routine. See page 46 for tips on what it might include.

Use your bed only for sleep or things that help you unwind (like physical intimacy or relaxing reading). If you watch a current events show in bed, your brain will associate bed with whatever bad news you saw, rather than with peaceful slumber.

STEP 1: Start with right bedtime. For most people, that's six to nine hours before they have to wake up in the morning.

STEP 2: Sleep well. If that's a challenge, look at my tips for happy sleep.

STEP 3: Wake up ready to share your joy with the world (or at least with your local barista).

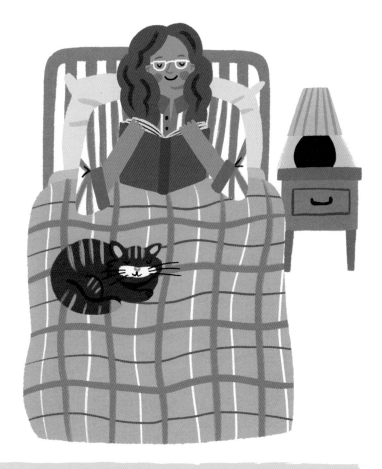

☐ If you got six to nine hours of sleep last night, or at least created the right environment for sleep, rest in victory.

MAKE A NIGHTTIME ROUTINE

Rituals offer meaning and regularity. When it comes to sleep, they have an extra benefit: They signal to your brain that it's time to switch off.

In your nighttime ritual, don't include high-intensity exercise, caffeine, or anything else that gets your blood pounding. Other than that, the most important thing is consistency. If you calmly sing the French national anthem to a stuffed duck every single night before bed, your brain will eventually associate it with sleep.

Just in case you don't want to learn "La Marseillaise," I've suggested some steps you might take. Don't feel pressured to do them all! As with all the tips in this book, take the ones that resonate with you. If some of them don't—well, don't lose any sleep over it.

STEP 1: Sometime before you get into bed, reflect on the events of your day. Be honest, but also kind to yourself. What did you accomplish that you're happy about? What could you have done better?

STEP 2: What outstanding issues from today still hang over you? Write down the steps you'll take to address them. This might not seem like a relaxing activity, but having a plan for unfinished business can reduce anxiety and obtrusive thoughts.

STEP 3: End your reflections on a positive note. This is a great time for gratitude journaling (page 122) or remembering funny things (page 21).

STEP 4: Stop looking at glowing screens at least an hour before bed. Otherwise, their light can disrupt your sleep cycle.

STEP 5: Begin winding down. A warm (not hot) bath will help your body reach ideal sleep temperature. A good book, peaceful music, or a soothing podcast can help put you in the right frame of mind. Gentle stretching exercises like yoga can help, too.

STEP 6: At roughly the same time every night, turn off the lights, close your eyes, and have a wonderful night's sleep.

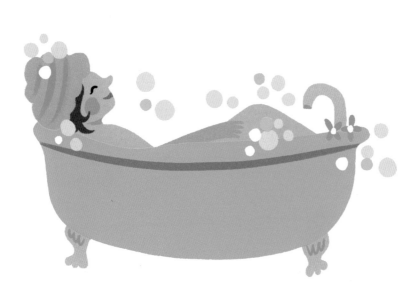

☐ If you've wound down with an evening ritual, tuck yourself in a warm blanket of success.

CHOOSE ONE PRESLEEP IMAGE

In the previous two entries, I suggested a couple of techniques to help you sleep. I thought this one deserved its own entry because (a) it's much less well known than the others, despite having been scientifically shown to be effective, and (b) it's a particularly relaxing way to work mindfulness into your daily routine.

STEP 1: Before you get in bed, choose an image that is pleasant *and* relaxing. It could be a calm, happy memory or a calm, happy fantasy. Think hanging out with a friend on a beautiful spring day, rather than blasting aliens.

STEP 2: As you lie down to sleep, call that image to mind. Ask yourself questions to engage your senses and your emotions. As you walked through that field, what did the flowers smell like? (Or, if it's a fantasy, what *would* they smell like?) How were you feeling (or would you feel) in that moment?

STEP 3: It's natural for your mind to wander to other thoughts. When you notice that happening, gently and without judgment redirect your attention back to your chosen image.

☐ If you used this technique to fall asleep, picture the happy image of a trophy.

NAP YOURSELF HAPPY

Justice never sleeps—but happiness certainly does. Afternoon naps have been shown to reduce your blood pressure, sharpen mental focus, and—you guessed it—boost happiness.

STEP 1: When you feel an afternoon lull, get in bed, or just put your head down on the desk. For many people, this will be somewhere between 11 AM and 4 PM. On average, aim for about six hours after you wake up that morning.

STEP 2: One study found maximum benefits from a mere ten minutes of dozing. Since people tend to lie awake for about ten minutes before drifting off, set an alarm for twenty minutes after you lie down. You can experiment with different nap lengths and see what feels best for you.

STEP 3: If you drink caffeine in the afternoon, try having your cup right *before* you lie down. You might find that it hits your blood just as your alarm goes off, letting you bounce right into action.

STEP 4: Doze.

STEP 5: Afterward, ease into wakefulness with two or three minutes of gentle stretching or walking.

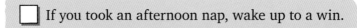 If you took an afternoon nap, wake up to a win.

SNAP OUT OF IT

Everybody has thoughts that make them unhappy. Sometimes you can eliminate them at their source—if you keep returning to an argument you had with a partner, it may be a sign you should talk to them about it.

But sometimes your brain grabs onto something unhelpful and won't let it go. It might be a specific memory you can't do anything about, like a dumb thing you said twenty years ago. Or it might be a pattern: a tendency to put yourself down or obsess about things you can't control. In those cases, you can use your body to distract your brain.

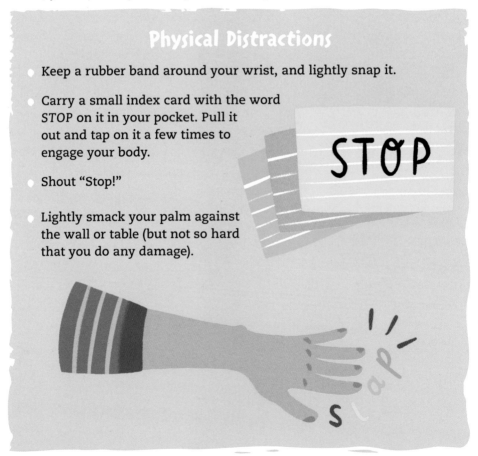

Physical Distractions

- Keep a rubber band around your wrist, and lightly snap it.

- Carry a small index card with the word STOP on it in your pocket. Pull it out and tap on it a few times to engage your body.

- Shout "Stop!"

- Lightly smack your palm against the wall or table (but not so hard that you do any damage).

STEP 1: Next time you find yourself dwelling on unhelpful thoughts, use one of the techniques on the previous page, or any other technique you find helpful, to interrupt them.

STEP 2: Focus your senses on something else. Run your hands on a nearby surface, pick up an object, or breathe through your nose and see if you can smell anything interesting.

STEP 3: If the thoughts just won't leave you alone, try writing them down. You can also set a specific time to think about them later.

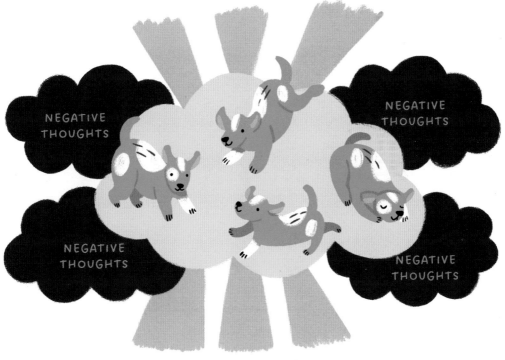

PUPPIES!

If you've used your body to distract your brain, give yourself a pat on the back.

EAT YOUR VEGETABLES

You know the stereotype of a glum health nut sadly shoveling vegetables into their face? Based on a review of forty-seven research findings, that's exactly backward. It turns out that, whatever your age, gender, or geographical location, there's a strong causal link between eating more than three portions of fruits and vegetables and happiness. Scientists are still figuring out why, but they think it goes beyond the fact that being healthy makes you happy. Could there be a specific micronutrient that boosts positive brain chemicals? Fortunately, you don't need to wait for an answer to make the power of plants work for you.

Tips for Enjoying Fruits and Vegetables

If you think "eating plants" is synonymous with "eating bland," fear not. It might take a little exploration, but you can find fruits and vegetables you'll love. Along the way, you'll rack up bonus happiness points by exploring somewhere new (page 119), learning something new (page 14), and eventually savoring the good stuff (page 34).

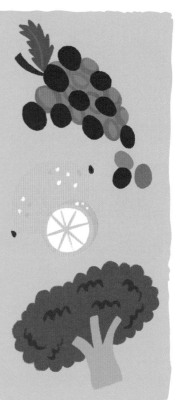

- Find out what's in season. Strawberries in spring are entirely different creatures from the flavorless red Ping-Pong balls you get in winter.

- Eat locally. The farther produce was shipped, the more likely it was selected for sturdiness over flavor.

- Try different varieties of the same plant. Compare apples to apples, and you might find you like the sweet Gala variety more than the tart Braeburn.

- Shop around. Some stores are just better at sourcing good-tasting produce. If you've got a local farmers' market, that's a great starting place— and even then, you might find you like some stalls more than others.

- Don't be afraid of frozen. Properly frozen produce can be more nutritious than once-fresh veggies that have sat around for too long.

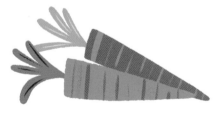

STEP 1: Eat one serving of your favorite fruit or vegetable. That's one medium-size fruit like an apple, half a big fruit like a grapefruit, one cup of leafy greens, or a half cup of chopped raw vegetables like carrots.

STEP 2: Repeat three or more times over the course of the day.

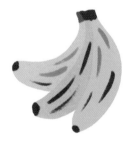

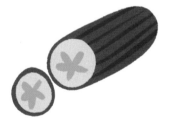

☐ If you've eaten more than three servings of fruit or vegetables today, consider it a victory dinner.

DRESS FOR THE MOOD YOU WANT, NOT THE MOOD YOU HAVE

One group took a test of mental focus while wearing a painter's smock. Another did it while wearing a doctor's jacket. The doctor's jacket group did better on the test.

And here's the twist: *They were the exact same garments.* The only difference was in how the researchers described them to the subjects.

The conclusion: How you think about your clothes can shape how you think. Psychologists call this phenomenon **enclothed cognition**. It's a relatively new topic of scientific study, but it's old news to actors, who have long used costumes not merely to convey their characters to the audience but to shape how they themselves feel.

You may already dress more cheerfully when you're feeling happy. But it may work the other way around as well. Putting on clothes you associate with good moods could actually induce those moods.

STEP 1: Think about how you would like to feel today.

STEP 2: Ask yourself: What clothes do you associate with the mood you want?

STEP 3: Dress for the mood you want— not the mood you have.

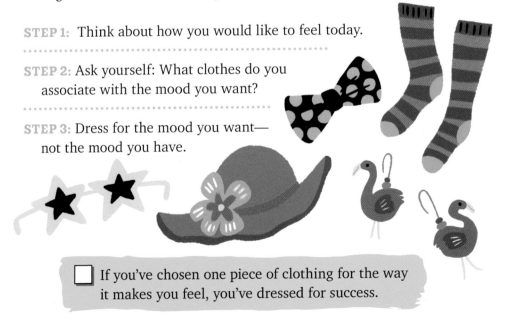

☐ If you've chosen one piece of clothing for the way it makes you feel, you've dressed for success.

DO IT LESS, ENJOY IT MORE

When I first moved to Los Angeles, I marveled at the sunshine every time I walked outside. A year later, I barely noticed it.

I was suffering from **hedonic adaptation**—the human tendency to get used to good things, forcing us to seek ever-newer pleasures.

Appropriately enough, another name for hedonic adaptation is the **hedonic treadmill**. Fortunately, there is a way to hop off.

If you've watched the TV show *Survivor*, you've seen contestants obsess over a single slice of not-very-appetizing pizza. In ordinary life, that slice would barely move their happiness needle. But after a week of living off rice and the occasional snail, even the mankiest combination of cheese, tomato, and dough makes their hearts sing.

You can create the same effect in your own life, and you don't have to eat snails to do it.

STEP 1: Think of something you do regularly that isn't as pleasurable as it once was.

STEP 2: Choose how long you'll do without it. Make it long enough to notice the absence. In one study, going even a week without chocolate enhanced people's pleasure when they started up again.

STEP 3: When your chosen time has passed, try it again.

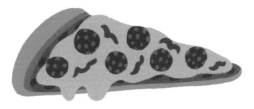

If you've passed up a routine pleasure, or reenjoyed a pleasure after taking some time off from it, now is the time to give yourself the win.

MOVE YOUR BUTT

You've heard it a million times: Exercise is good for you. If being reminded to exercise counted as exercise, you'd be an Olympic athlete. But here are some things you might not know:

- Long-term exercise can rewire your brain to have more available dopamine receptors, making you literally more able to feel joy.

- Short-term exercise can boost your happiness, even in tiny amounts. As little as ten extra minutes a day significantly improves your odds of being in a good mood.

- There's no one form of exercise it has to be—a stretching and balancing exercise like yoga is as psychologically effective as an all-out sprint.

To be clear, sweaty exertion has substantial physical benefits, and your doctor probably has an opinion about how much you should do for optimum body health. But as your personal happiness advisor, all I care about is that you do *something*.

STEP 1: Get moving. If you don't know what to do, check out the sidebar for some possibilities.

STEP 2: Keep moving for at least ten minutes.

STEP 3: If you're having fun, keep going beyond that. As long as you listen to your body and avoid injury, exercise is one mind-altering drug you're not going to overdose on.

All of These Count as Exercise

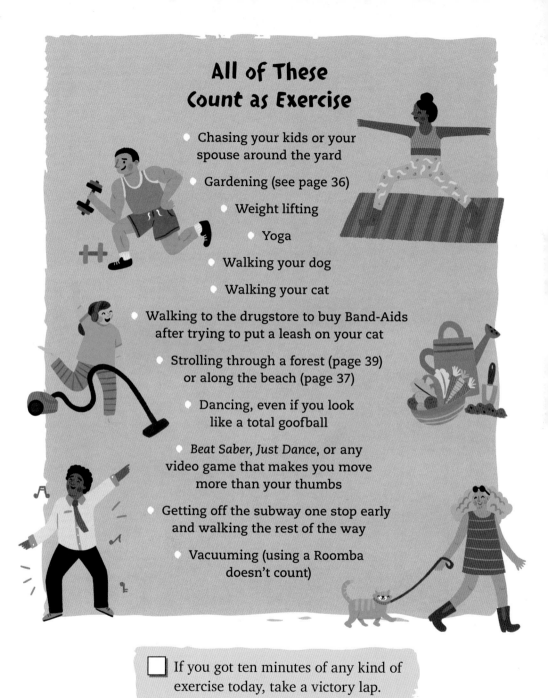

- Chasing your kids or your spouse around the yard
- Gardening (see page 36)
- Weight lifting
- Yoga
- Walking your dog
- Walking your cat
- Walking to the drugstore to buy Band-Aids after trying to put a leash on your cat
- Strolling through a forest (page 39) or along the beach (page 37)
- Dancing, even if you look like a total goofball
- *Beat Saber*, *Just Dance*, or any video game that makes you move more than your thumbs
- Getting off the subway one stop early and walking the rest of the way
- Vacuuming (using a Roomba doesn't count)

☐ If you got ten minutes of any kind of exercise today, take a victory lap.

FEED YOUR GUT

Your gut is its own ecosystem, filled with so many bacteria, yeasts, and fungi that if you could put them on a scale, they'd weigh more than your brain. Scientists are in the early days of studying the gut microbiome, but preliminary evidence suggests that it might play a role in mental health.

Based on where the science stands as of this writing, don't spend money on supplements. But if you have a normal immune system, there's no drawback to including gut-healthy foods in a balanced diet—and there might be a real happiness-boosting benefit.

STEP 1: Eat a probiotic food—that's one with live, healthy bacteria in it. Yogurt, kombucha, and sauerkraut are common examples. Fermented foods can sometimes be processed in a way that kills the healthy bacteria before it reaches your insides, so check the label for phrases like "live, active cultures" or "probiotic."

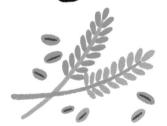

STEP 2: Eat a prebiotic food—that's one rich in fiber that you can't digest but your microbiome can. These tend to be high-fiber foods like whole grain oats, apples, or berries. Think of Step 1 as planting a garden and Step 2 as watering it.

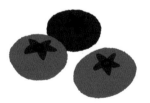
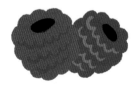

If you ate one gut-healthy meal today, gobble up a win.

SMILE, DARN YA, SMILE

One of my pet peeves is when grown-ups tell sad children, "Come on, smile." I've always felt that if you're sad, you should cry. In many ways, psychologists agree: Suppressing negative emotions can have serious long-term consequences for your mental health. Sometimes you just need to let yourself be miserable (page 108).

But there's scientific evidence that forcing a smile makes you feel temporarily happy. In other words, what you feel shapes your expressions—but your expressions may shape how you feel. Psychologists call this the **facial feedback hypothesis**.

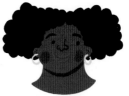

To be clear, for long-term happiness and mental health, it's important to acknowledge your sad emotions. But if you want a quick pick-me-up . . . well, come on. Smile!

STEP 1: Smile.

STEP 2: Pay attention to how it makes you feel. Are you a little happier? Can you feel your forced smile becoming more genuine? If so, let the genuine smile linger. If not, don't force yourself to feel things you simply don't feel.

STEP 3: Use this technique when you need a quick emotional boost—but don't substitute it for acknowledging and dealing with your negative emotions.

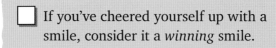

☐ If you've cheered yourself up with a smile, consider it a *winning* smile.

RENAME THOSE BUTTERFLIES

Which comes first: your anxiety or that jittery feeling in your stomach? You might think the emotion leads and the body follows, but it's not quite that simple.

According to **appraisal theory**, we judge our own emotions based, at least in part, on how our bodies react to outside stimuli. In a classic study, volunteers were injected with a stimulant. Some were warned it could make their hearts beat faster, and some weren't. Then each volunteer was placed in a room with a stooge—a person in cahoots with the researcher—who acted either euphoric or furious.

Those in a room with a euphoric stooge were more likely to act euphoric, and those stuck with a furious stooge were more likely to become angry themselves. But the group that knew about the stimulant's cardiac side effect were less likely to catch the stooge's mood. Apparently, if you feel your heart pounding and you don't know why, your brain will cast around for an explanation. In this case, the volunteers not warned about the side effect of the stimulant used the emotion expressed by the stooge to "explain" their rapid heartbeats. And if your brain concludes that you must be feeling a certain emotion . . . then, by God, you feel that emotion.

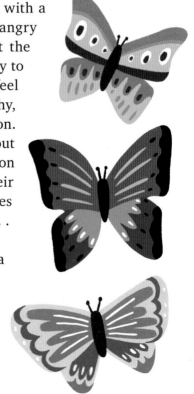

In another study, men approached by a female researcher on a rickety suspension bridge were more likely to flirt with her than men approached on a more stable, less scary bridge. It's surprisingly easy to mistake a heart pounding from fear for one pounding from love.

Even if you don't want to take your next date to a rickety suspension bridge, you can use this information to your advantage. Through **cognitive reappraisal**, you can reinterpret your own reactions in a way that makes you happier.

STEP 1: Next time you're feeling anxious, notice and label the physical symptoms, like a rapidly beating heart.

STEP 2: Remember that those are the same symptoms as excitement. Think about what you might be excited about. If you're about to give an important speech before a big crowd, you might be excited about the opportunity to reach so many people.

STEP 3: Say "I'm excited!" out loud.

☐ If you've used cognitive reappraisal, appraise that as a victory.

REACH OUT AND TOUCH SOMEONE

Sometimes what scientists discover when they apply the most advanced scientific methods to human cognition is this:

We're basically a bunch of apes.

If you've seen a documentary on apes, you know they spend hours grooming one another—as much as 15 percent of their day. It's not because it takes that long to pick off a few nits. It's because primates need to touch and be touched.

In our particular species of hairless apes, positive touches release oxytocin, a trust-promoting hormone. Just holding hands with a loved one can make your body react less negatively to stress.

Touch is even its own language—research shows that people can distinguish between touches that communicate compassion, love, or fear.

So reach out and touch somebody, no matter how nit-free you are.

STEP 1: Find a situation in which physical touch is appropriate. Cuddle with a toddler, politely shake a colleague's hand, or book an appointment with a massage therapist.

STEP 2: Touch or be touched, as appropriate.

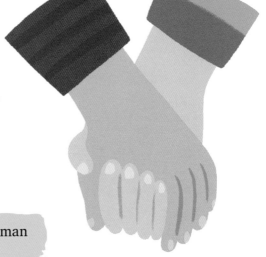

☐ If you've touched another human today, give yourself the win.

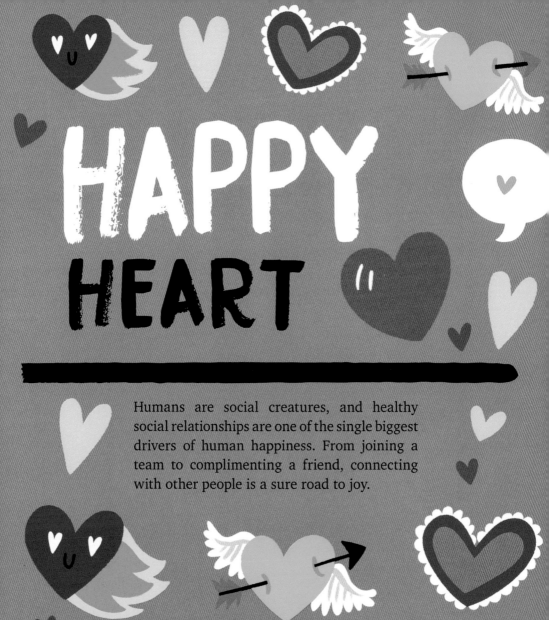

HAPPY
HEART

Humans are social creatures, and healthy social relationships are one of the single biggest drivers of human happiness. From joining a team to complimenting a friend, connecting with other people is a sure road to joy.

JOIN THE TEAM

As I said on page 56, any exercise makes you happier than no exercise. But exercising as part of a team will make you happiest of all. In a study comparing women who worked out on their own to women who joined a sports club to work out, both groups were in equally good shape. Both groups were more satisfied with their lives than the average nonexercising population. But the *most* satisfied group? You guessed it: the folks on a team. Researchers suspect it's because they were combining the happy-making power of exercise with the uplifting boost of social interaction.

Joining a team probably won't result in gold medals or multimillion-dollar endorsements. But it may make you feel as if you're winning at life.

STEP 1: Think about a sport you enjoy. You don't have to be great at it!

STEP 2: Find a club in your area that's roughly on your level. Try contacting your local gym, or just type "(YOUR SPORT) club" into a search engine.

STEP 3: Show up for practice, do your best, and have fun. If the team is too high-pressure or competitive for your tastes, keep looking!

☐ If you've practiced with a team or sports club (or even signed up to join one), give yourself the win, even if your team lost.

GET SWEATY WITH A FRIEND

If joining a team is more of a commitment than you're willing to make right now, you can still combine the benefits of exercise and social interaction. And you may set off a virtuous circle: Exercising releases endorphins, as does synchronizing movements with another human, and endorphins enhance social bonding. Meanwhile, the pleasure of social interaction can help you ignore fatigue and work out longer than you otherwise would.

Based on current research, the faster you get your heart going, the stronger the resulting bonds. Music, too, seems to increase bonding, making a high-intensity dance class the ultimate social experience. But whether you're jazzercising or just strolling through the woods, doing it with a friend can make you happier.

STEP 1: Take an exercise class with other people, or recruit a buddy to join you for a run, a brisk walk, or a Ping-Pong match.

STEP 2: Enjoy the companionship and the happy glow.

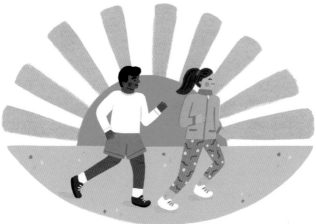

☐ If you've exercised with another person today, give yourself the win.

ADD MORE HAPPY TO YOUR HOLIDAYS

One Thanksgiving when I was little, my mom and dad and their friends Cora and Marty told a mildly amusing story about a trip they took in a car with a broken windshield wiper. The next year, they told the same story, which annoyed all the kids at the table, which, of course, motivated our parents to subject us to the exact same story the *next* year, which prompted my generation to do everything we could to interrupt it. By the time I was a teenager, the Windshield Wiper Story had evolved into an elaborate ritual that took up most of Thanksgiving dinner.

My teenage self would never admit it, but my parents and their friends were on to something, and science has finally caught up. A series of studies with nearly one thousand participants found that having a family ritual on a holiday is associated with having a closer family—and, therefore, a happier holiday. Objectively speaking, Thanksgiving plus turkey is good, but Thanksgiving plus turkey plus windshield wipers is even better.

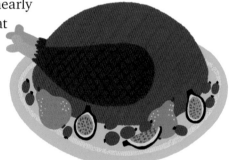

STEP 1: Find a holiday. If there's not one coming up soon enough, invent one. In my household, we celebrate the birthday of Ruth Graves Wakefield, inventor of the chocolate chip cookie. (June 17, in case you're wondering. See the sidebar for other suggestions.)

STEP 2: Add a ritual to it that involves the whole family. This might be a brand-new ritual or an extension of an existing one onto another day. Just make sure you involve at least one other person, if not the whole family; solo rituals don't seem to have the same positive effect.

Holidays You Might Not Know About

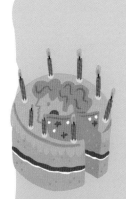

January 8: Elvis Presley's Birthday

First Saturday in February: National Take Your Child to the Library Day

March 14: Pi Day

April 10: National Siblings Day

May 12: National Limerick Day

Last Saturday in June: Great American Picnic Day

July 1: International Joke Day

August 30: Birthday of Mary Shelley, author of *Frankenstein*

September 19: International Talk like a Pirate Day

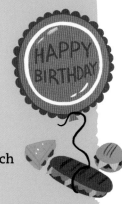

October 1: World Vegetarian Day

November 13: Birthday of John Montagu, Earl of Sandwich, who invented the sandwich

December 16: Beethoven's Birthday

 If you've observed one ritual with your loved ones, or thought about how to do so on a future holiday, give yourself the win.

UNFRIEND SOCIAL MEDIA

Relationships are a major component of happiness. Social media is all about relationships. Therefore, social media should increase happiness.

Unfortunately, it doesn't seem to work that way.

Social media use has been correlated with increased feelings of envy and increased risk of depression. In one experiment, people who deactivated Facebook in the month before a big election reported improved moods, plus an hour of extra free time a day.

It may depend on how you use social media. One study showed that people's well-being increased when they got direct personal messages from friends, but not when they got "likes" or just read public status updates.

Social media is a brand-new phenomenon, and science is still catching up with it. One day, there will be an RDA for clicking "like." In the meantime, why not experiment on yourself?

STEP 1: Take a full twenty-four hours off from social media. No Facebook, no Instagram, no whatever-has-been-invented-since-you-started-reading-this-sentence-but-will-be-bankrupt-by-the-end-of-the-page.

STEP 2: Use the time to make direct contact with a close friend. It's fine if you send them an email or an instant message. The point isn't that electronics are evil—it's just that direct personal messages are better than broadcasts to the world.

STEP 3: At the end of the twenty-four hours, check in with yourself. Did making direct contact feel better than clicking "like"? How do you want to balance your use of social media going forward?

☐ If you've taken time off from social media and used it to make direct contact with someone, make direct contact with victory.

HIDE YOUR PHONE

My kids don't believe me when I tell them this, but once upon a time, people used their phones to talk to each other—nothing more, nothing less. Their only reason for existence was social connection.

Nowadays, smartphones can be used for all sorts of reasons, some of which bring us together and many of which don't. Obviously, playing *Candy Crush Saga* when your partner is trying to talk to you isn't good for your relationship. But studies have shown that just having your phone visible during a conversation reduces feelings of closeness, trust, and empathy. Apparently, the mere sight of your personal *Candy Crush* machine is enough to start some corner of your brain thinking about *Candy Crush* (or whatever your personal addiction is).

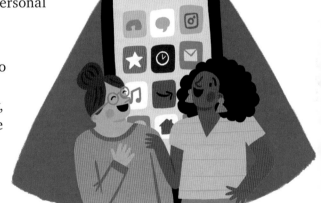

STEP 1: Next time you want to have a high-quality social interaction with somebody, put your phone somewhere you can't see or feel it.

☐ If you've removed the distraction of your phone for a social interaction, consider that a victory.

SHARE YOUR SUCCESSES

Celebrations can release endorphins, your brain's feel-good chemical, making you feel good now. They reinforce good habits, setting you up for future successes. And turning a celebration into a party bonds you with everybody there, reinforcing the relationships that form one of the Felicitous Four. Throw in some dancing for extra bonding power, plus all the good things that exercise brings. Whether it's a massive shindig or a party of two, you'll be serving up a multilayer dip of good feelings.

STEP 1: Identify a recent success, whether it's huge (like finishing that novel) or tiny (like making your bed as soon as you got up).

STEP 2: Invite one or more friends to celebrate with you in person, on the phone, or online.

STEP 3: Celebrate in style— *your* style. Whether that involves Dom Pérignon with a thousand of your friends or a quiet cup of tea with just one of them is up to you.

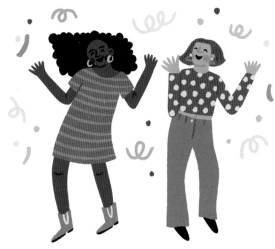

☐ If you've celebrated at least one success with at least one friend, celebrate *this* success.

MAKE A FRIEND DOWN THE BLOCK

For twenty years, psychologists tracked 4,739 volunteers in Massachusetts. They discovered something amazing: 4,739 people were willing to be tracked for twenty years.

Equally amazing, when they mapped social relationships among the volunteers, psychologists could track happiness or unhappiness as it flowed among friends. Joy, it turns out, is a public health condition.

And some relationships spread joy more effectively than others. A spouse you live with is more likely to give it to you than a sibling who lives far away. And you know who's more likely to give it to you than either of those? A friend who lives within a mile of you.

Why would a local friend's mood affect yours more than a spouse's mood would? Perhaps your spouse is better at making you happy even when they're miserable.

Another possible explanation: Research shows that moods are more transmittable within the same gender, and none of the participants in this study had same-gender marriages. Whatever the reason, you can seed your own happiness network by bringing joy to people near you.

STEP 1: If you're close enough to somebody in your neighborhood to reach out to them, then give them a call, drop them a friendly email, or do something else to make them happy.

· ·

STEP 2: If you don't have a local friend, take a step to make one. Organize a block party, arrange a playdate, or volunteer locally.

☐ If you've reached out to one person who lives within a mile of you, consider that a local victory.

HAVE HAPPY,
WELL-CONNECTED FRIENDS

Although the study I talked about on page 71 put special emphasis on having local friendships, it also found something more broadly applicable: Happiness spreads through social networks more strongly than sadness. That means that people who function as the hub of a network—the ones who seem to know *everybody*—end up at the center of a lot more positive emotions than negative ones.

STEP 1: Think about the happiest friend you've got. If you've got lots of happy friends, zero in on the one who seems to know everybody.

STEP 2: Reach out to them in the most direct way you can. Being in the same place is the best way, but if that's not possible, a videoconference, a phone call, or even an email will do. (Of course, if your usually-happy friend is feeling lousy, let them feel lousy! See page 108 for more on the value of acknowledging bad moods.)

STEP 3: Happiness spreads both ways. Next time you're in a great mood, think about a friend who *doesn't* have a huge social network. Pay it forward by reaching out to them and sharing your joy.

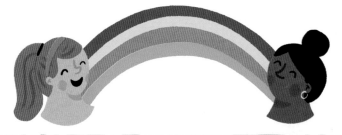

☐ If you've reached out to a happy, well-connected friend or shared your own happiness with a friend today, give yourself the win.

SHARE THE INTELLECTUAL WEALTH

Learning a new thing makes you happy (page 14). Doing something good for a friend or loved one makes you happy (page 93). Teach a friend something new and you make both of you happy.

You also bring the two of you closer together. Studies of marriages show that romantic couples are happier and more stable when they each contribute to the other's *self-expansion*, or acquisition of new knowledge and experiences. It seems likely that the same applies to nonromantic relationships as well.

STEP 1: Find an interesting fact that your friend or romantic partner doesn't know or a skill you can teach them.

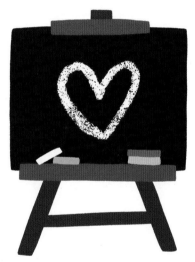

STEP 2: Think about whether it's something this particular person would be interested in learning.

STEP 3: Share it!

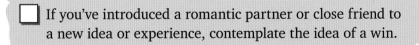

☐ If you've introduced a romantic partner or close friend to a new idea or experience, contemplate the idea of a win.

BE LESS STRAIGHT WITH YOUR PARTNER

People with same-sex spouses are less stressed and more satisfied than people married to the opposite sex*. Obviously, I'm not advising that my fellow straights marry people they're not attracted to. But it's worth reflecting on what we're doing wrong.

At least in part, it comes down to this: A couple with two men or two women can't fall into the trap of assigning roles based on gender. For example, half of gay couples share laundry duties equally, while only a third of straight couples do. Straight couples are more likely to hand the bulk of child care to the woman; gay couples have to figure out which division actually makes everybody the happiest. Straight men are more likely to speak harshly to their romantic partners than gay men or women would.

(*Side note: I'm speaking in binary terms about men and women because I haven't found equivalent research on couples with one or more nonbinary partners.)

STEP 1: If you want to marry somebody of the same gender, go ahead and do it. Otherwise, skip to Step 2.

STEP 2: Think about your relationships, romantic or otherwise, with the opposite sex. What is the division of labor in them? That can include emotional labor (like asking about the other person's feelings) as well as household chores. Is the woman in the relationship doing more of the work? How would the relationship be different if you were both the same gender and couldn't fall back on stereotypical divisions of labor? Would you both end up happier?

STEP 3: Next time you have a disagreement with a member of the opposite sex, notice your tone. Would you speak differently if you were talking to a same-sex friend?

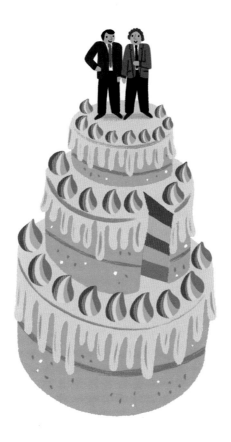

☐ If you've distributed roles in an important relationship based on happiness or fairness rather than gender, give yourself the win.

LEARN A FAMILY STORY

Pride in your family heritage can be a strong source of individual identity and meaning. And storytelling is a vital method of transmitting that heritage.

You can take a pretty relaxed attitude toward most of the tips in this book, but this one comes with a ticking clock. Your oldest family stories are stored in the minds of your relatives with the least time left on this earth. To paraphrase Amadou Hampâté Bâ: When an old person dies, it's like a library burning to the ground. I'd encourage you to use this tip while as many libraries as possible are still standing.

Conversation Starters

- Is there a story that makes you proud of our family?

- What's the earliest thing you remember personally?

- How far back do you know about our family history? What do you know about our ancestors?

- Can you tell me any stories about [a family member you are both close to]?

- How did you meet your spouse?

- What family traditions do you know of? How do you think they started?

STEP 1: Think about the oldest family member whose memory is still intact. (If you *are* the oldest family member, skip to Step 4.)

STEP 2: Visit them in person, or call them, and start them talking about family history. If you're not sure how to begin, see the sidebar for some suggestions.

STEP 3: If possible, record your conversation and share it with other family members.

STEP 4: If you know any good family stories yourself, share them with your loved ones.

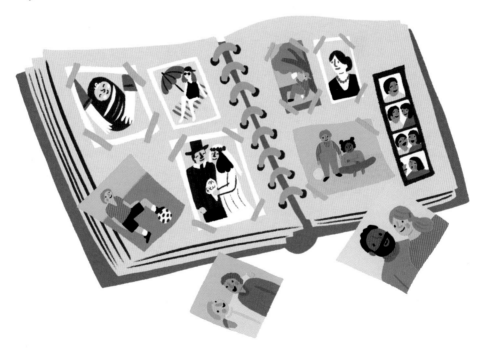

☐ If you've learned one new family story, or helped pass on one that you already knew, tell yourself the tale of your triumph.

SEND AN SOS TO AN OSO

We all know what the perfect relationship looks like. It's when one person fulfills every single need you have. Who wouldn't want a partner who can cheer you up when you're sad, enhance your joy when you're happy, and entertain you when you're bored, all while making a soufflé and walking your dog?

It turns out there's a problem with that model (beyond the obvious difficulty of whisking eggs while holding a leash).

Yes, having somebody who can help you manage your moods is healthy. Psychologists have even coined a word for a relationship that helps you regulate your emotions: **emotionship**.

But it turns out that people with multiple emotionships are better off than those who rely on a single one. Even if you're lucky enough to have a multitalented significant other, there are going to be some situations they handle better than others. That's why you need an Other Significant Other, or OSO.

Turning to an OSO doesn't just help you. It can help relieve the relationship pressure of expecting an SO to do things they're just not suited for.

STEP 1: Think about the people you're close to. Are some of them better in certain situations than others? If you have a primary romantic partner, are there moods they're less able to help you with?

STEP 2: If you don't have a close friend who feels right for any particular mood, think about your casual friends who might be good in that situation. What can you do to strengthen that friendship now so they'll be there for you when you need them?

STEP 3: Reach out to the right emotionship for the emotions you're feeling now.

STEP 4: If you have a primary romantic partner, make sure you stay connected with them. You want to grow your relationship with your OSO—not shrink your relationship with your SO.

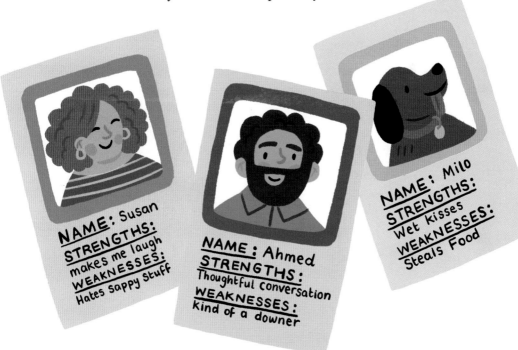

NAME: Susan
STRENGTHS: makes me laugh
WEAKNESSES: Hates sappy stuff

NAME: Ahmed
STRENGTHS: Thoughtful conversation
WEAKNESSES: kind of a downer

NAME: Milo
STRENGTHS: Wet kisses
WEAKNESSES: Steals Food

☐ If you've reached out to the right emotionship, or laid the groundwork to do so, give yourself the win.

BE SOCIALLY OPTIMISTIC

Here's an interesting correlation vs. causation conundrum:

Being confident that people will like you is correlated with being liked. But which way does it go? Does confidence make you popular, or does popularity make you confident?

Research suggests that it goes both ways. By entering a social interaction with a feeling of confidence, you increase the odds of it going well. That will make you more confident about the next interaction. And since "positive relationships" is one of the Felicitous Four, you'll be on a self-fulfilling road to happiness.

If you find it hard to start that cycle, there's some encouraging news. One study showed that no matter how nervous you feel, thinking about the other person's nervousness can make you more confident.

STEP 1: Next time you're meeting somebody new, remind yourself that they're meeting somebody new, too. Think about the fact that they're probably a little nervous, even if they don't show it.

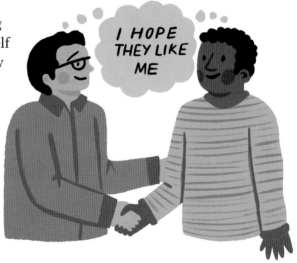

STEP 2: Picture yourself as a host, putting a nervous guest at ease with a warm greeting.

☐ If you've approached a social interaction with optimism, say "Hello" to victory.

INDULGE IN NOSTALGIA

As far as positive emotions go, nostalgia doesn't get enough respect. For many of us, there's a faint whiff of embarrassment about the word—a hint that, in appreciating the past, we're shortchanging the present.

Certainly, nostalgia is unhealthy when it leads to bitterness. But over the past two decades, evidence has emerged that nostalgia can be a healthy coping mechanism for the disappointments of life. It can boost your mood and provide meaning, while bonding you closer with friends.

STEP 1: Remember a good time you had with a friend or family member.

STEP 2: Reach out to your loved one and reminisce about the good time together. Talk about not just the events but what made them meaningful to you.

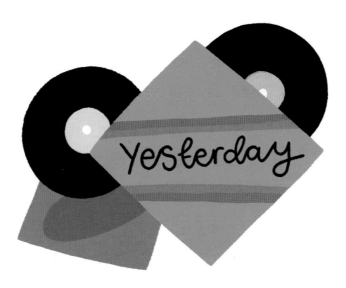

☐ If you've bonded nostalgically with a friend today, look back on it in triumph.

WHAT A CLEVER READER YOU ARE!

Of course you know that it feels good to receive compliments. Somebody as perceptive as you figured that out long ago. But did you know that *giving* compliments also makes you happier, according to an ingenious experiment by some absolutely delightful scientists?

No joke: Writing that paragraph, as silly as it was, made me grin like an idiot. Think how good it will feel to give an actual compliment to a real person you know.

STEP 1: Think of a specific thing you enjoy, respect, or admire about somebody in your life.

STEP 2: Tell that person how you feel.

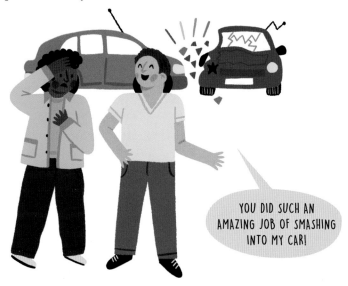

YOU DID SUCH AN AMAZING JOB OF SMASHING INTO MY CAR!

☐ If you've paid a heartfelt compliment, compliment yourself on a victory.

FORGIVE SOMEBODY'S TRESPASSES

> "The weak never forgive.
> Forgiveness is the attribute of the strong."
> —Mahatma Gandhi

Philosophers have understood the power of forgiveness for centuries, but it's only recently that psychologists have begun to quantify it. They've found that people more willing to forgive show greater life satisfaction and improved well-being.

The more committed your relationship is to the transgressor, the more your psychological well-being improves when you forgive them. One study found that a tendency to forgive one's spouse was more strongly associated with happiness than a tendency to forgive people in general.

Importantly, I'm talking about forgiving nontraumatic wrongs. If you've suffered something traumatic, I'd encourage you to talk with a professional therapist (page 134) about what role forgiveness should play in your healing process.

STEP 1: Make a conscious decision to forgive somebody who has wronged you. Just making the choice to forgive can make you happier, even if you feel as if you haven't forgiven them completely.

STEP 2: If they've apologized to you, reach out and let them know that you accept their apology. Remember: Even when you forgive somebody, you're allowed to lay out clear expectations for their behavior in the future.

> ☐ If you've chosen to forgive one friend
> or loved one, give yourself the win.

SING YOUR HEART OUT

Despite what you've seen in any behind-the-scenes rock documentary, singing together is a major source of good feelings. In fact, a review of over sixty studies found that music and singing enhances happiness while reducing or even preventing depression.

Scientists are still figuring out the mechanism by which social singing works its magic, but perhaps, like dancing and concertgoing (page 128), it combines self-expression with social interaction.

The best part is that singing ability doesn't seem to matter. Whether you sing like an angel or a hungover garbage disposal, you can still boost your happiness by singing together. Just stay away from the documentary cameras and don't smash anybody's guitar, and you'll be fine.

STEP 1: Whether you join a formal choir or belt out off-key show tunes with your roommate while you do the dishes, find an opportunity to sing with another human being.

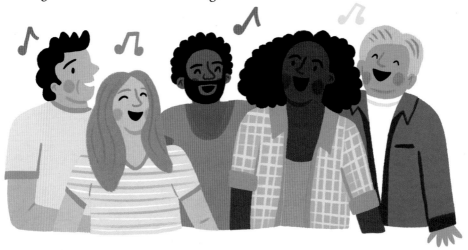

☐ If you've sung with one other person, sing a song of triumph.

STEAL HAPPINESS OFF
A FRIEND'S PLATE

When researchers asked 8,250 British adults about their sense of well-being, and then looked for correlations with various aspects of their life, some results weren't surprising. The biggest predictor of unhappiness was having a mental illness. The third-biggest predictor was being "very dissatisfied" with your love life.

But the second predictor of misery was more unexpected: always eating alone.

Let me add two grains of salt to this scientific meal. First, as ever, correlation is not causation. Eating alone might make you miserable—or maybe miserable people just don't want company. Second, the study was sponsored by a grocery store chain. I'm not saying that sinister-looking checkout clerks paid a midnight visit to the researcher's house, ominously smacking cucumbers into their palms. I'm also not saying they didn't.

Caveats aside, this is another case where science and your grandmother agree: Come over, grab a plate, and have a chat.

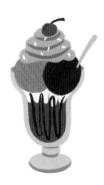

STEP 1: Get together with a friend.

STEP 2: Eat food. Avoid distractions like phones or TV screens.

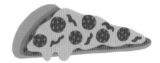

☐ If you've eaten with another person, enjoy the taste of victory.

MAKE A SOCIAL PLAN

This year, for the first time in decades, I made a New Year's resolution. I had given them up because they never seemed to improve my life. But in researching this book, I found a study that finally told me what I was doing wrong.

German researchers asked more than 1,500 volunteers how satisfied they were with their life and what they planned to do in the coming year to make it better. (I assume that in German, the entire question was a single word.) Then, a year later, the researchers followed up to see who was actually happier with their lot. Only one group felt better off:

The people who had planned to have more social interaction.

You don't need to wait until December 31 to learn from their experience.

STEP 1: Come up with a way you can become more socially engaged over the next twelve months. Will you join a bowling league? Call friends more often? Throw a monthly dinner party?

....

STEP 2: Consider whether there's a second, related goal that would support the first (see sidebar). Will you be more likely to have friends over for dinner if you finally finish unpacking the plates from your move last year?

Co-Action Plan

Believe it or not, two resolutions are sometimes easier to keep than one. When two goals support each other, psychologists call this *co-action*. For example, you might resolve to use your phone for Twitter less often and for calling your friends more often.

STEP 3: Get out your calendar and put the specific steps you'll need to take on the right days. If you're throwing a dinner party, how far in advance will you need to send out the invitations? To pick a menu? To buy a soufflé dish and/or a fire extinguisher, depending on how handy you are with a stove? If the preparation for your goal seems overwhelming, go for something simpler; the important thing is to socialize.

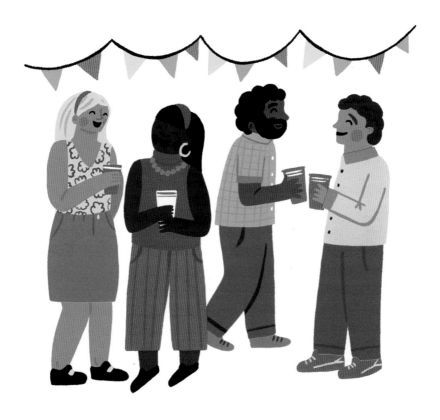

☐ If you've come up with a plan to be more social, give yourself the win.

TALK TO STRANGERS

A wizard casts a spell on you. From now on, whenever you're in public, you've got to chat with at least one stranger. Is the wizard's spell a blessing or a curse?

Most people would say "curse." And most people would be wrong.

In a Chicago study, commuters were randomly asked either to strike up a conversation with a stranger on their train journey or to sit silently. The conversation group wasn't happy about it: They predicted that talking to a stranger would make their commute less productive and less pleasant. Surveyed afterward, the conversation group was happier than the silent one—and the two groups had equally productive commutes.

It turns out that even grumpy commuters need human contact. Who knew (other than any psychologist who has ever studied human behavior)?

STEP 1: Next time you're out in the world, keep an eye out for a stranger who has a few minutes to chat. Maybe it'll be the person sitting next to you on the subway train or the clerk in an otherwise empty shop.

STEP 2: Offer them a conversation starter beyond a perfunctory, "How are you?" Ask them how their day is going, in a tone that makes it clear you really want to know. Or ask if they did anything interesting over the weekend. Or tell them something funny you saw recently.

STEP 3: If they're reluctant to talk, let the conversation drop. If not, keep it going for as long as you both enjoy it. Here's a trick my mom taught me: When somebody tells you what they do, you can always respond, "You must have some fascinating stories," and it will turn out to be true. Everybody has stories. Most people just never get asked for them.

☐ If you've struck up a conversation with one stranger today, give yourself the win.

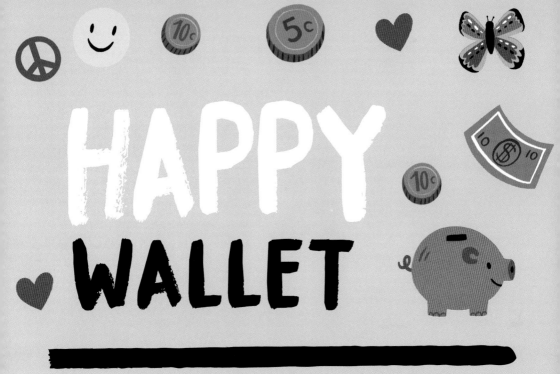

HAPPY
WALLET

Contrary to popular opinion, money can buy happiness, but only when it's spent very carefully on the right things. If you have some cash to spare, then this section will help you get the maximum happiness bang for your buck.

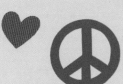
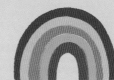
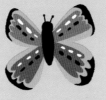

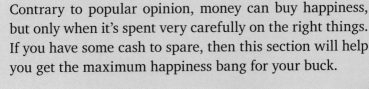

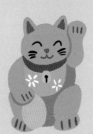

PAY DOWN DEBT

On the issue of debt, economists and happiness experts display a rare unanimity: High-interest consumer debt—whether it's a payday loan or an unpaid credit card bill—stinks. People with more consumer debt are more stressed and more depressed. They're more anxious about *everything*, not just the money they owe. Debt interferes with sleep, relationships, and enjoying the moment, which makes it a one-man anti–Felicitous Four.

STEP 1: Practice self-compassion. You aren't the only person to fall into debt. And you won't be the only person to work your way out of it.

STEP 2: Ask yourself if you have any spare money you can use right now to pay down your debt, even a little.

STEP 3: Think through a budget. The average American could eliminate their credit card debt within a year if they could devote 15 percent of their monthly earnings to paying it down. Can you set aside that much each month to pay down your debt? Cut expenses, but leave space for occasional treats that will help you enjoy life. That will make it easier to stick with your plan.

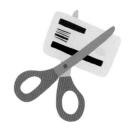

STEP 4: A nonprofit credit counselor can help you consider all the options, including declaring bankruptcy. You can find one through your local credit union, religious organization, or nonprofit agency. Make sure your counselor is accredited through the National Foundation for Credit Counseling or the Financial Counseling Association of America. You can find more information at **usa.gov/debt**

☐ If you've created a budget, consulted a professional, or taken other steps to get your high-interest debt under control, give yourself the win.

KILL ZOMBIE COSTS

Whether you want to reduce debt (page 90) or buy time (page 97), cutting back expenses can be painful. An easy place to start is with zombie costs—recurring payments for stuff you no longer use.

Like the zombies in any good postapocalyptic tale, zombie costs seem to be multiplying. Decades ago, the only things you subscribed to were magazines, and possibly a gym. Now you could be paying a monthly fee for software you don't use or a streaming service you never watch.

Of course, if you get pleasure, meaning, or utility out of a subscription, it can be a fun way to pay now and enjoy later (page 100). The point isn't to make you doubt purchases you're happy with. It's to plug small financial leaks.

STEP 1: Review your credit and debit card statements. Look for subscription fees and other recurring payments you're no longer getting something out of.

STEP 2: Take the time to cancel whatever it is.

STEP 3: Calculate how much the fee adds up to every year, and spend that on something that makes you happy. If you need inspiration, just read the rest of this chapter!

☐ If you've identified and eliminated one zombie cost, compliment yourself on your braaaaaaains.

GIVE IT AWAY, GIVE IT AWAY, GIVE IT AWAY NOW

Two groups of research participants got cash and instructions on how to spend it. One group got five dollars, and the other twenty dollars. Which recipients reported the most happiness?

The ones who were told to spend it on other people.

People who kept twenty dollars were no happier than people who kept five dollars. But people who spent the money on somebody else were happiest of all, no matter the amount.

Similarly, surveys show that once you can afford the necessities of life, income level doesn't have a huge effect on happiness. But whatever people's income is, those who spend a higher percentage of it on **pro-social spending** are happiest.

STEP 1: Find a charity that you, personally, think will make the world a better place. You might also consider a close friend or family member who could use some financial support (see page 93).

STEP 2: Give money to that good cause.

STEP 3: For an ongoing boost, decide how much money you're comfortable donating over the course of a year, then sign up for a monthly donation. Getting a regular reminder of the good you're doing will brighten your entire year.

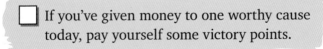

☐ If you've given money to one worthy cause today, pay yourself some victory points.

BUY (A FRIEND'S) HAPPINESS

Giving to people in your life brings just as much happiness as giving to charity. And you maximize the positive effect on your mood by giving gifts you can enjoy together—treating a friend or family member to one shared spa day will make you happier than buying two spa days to enjoy alone.

The emotional closeness of the relationship seems to matter more than the type of relationship. Giving a gift to a favorite coworker you see every day will make you happier than giving a gift to an uncle you feel vaguely positive toward. (IMPORTANT: If my nephews and nieces are reading this, please skip the previous sentence.)

STEP 1: Identify some discretionary income you were going to spend on yourself.

STEP 2: Figure out a way to spend it on a friend, *with* a friend.

STEP 3: Make the gift. And if your friend offers to reciprocate some other time, let them. Don't they deserve happiness, too?

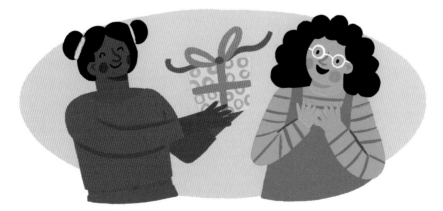

☐ If you've spent money on a friend today, you've just bought a victory.

BUY EXPERIENCES, NOT THINGS

If you spend $5,000 on diamond earrings, then wear them to an amazing show you paid twenty dollars to see, an economist might assume that the earrings were the best part of the night. If they weren't, why would the market have priced them so much higher?

A psychologist would know better.

Time and time again, studies show that money spent on experiences brings more happiness (and causes fewer regrets) than money spent on things. Maybe that's because things can break, rust, or become obsolete, but memories never do.

STEP 1: Identify a sum of money you plan on using for an object that isn't strictly necessary.

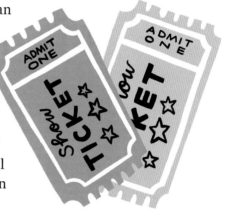

STEP 2: Find an experience you can buy for that sum instead. Bonus points if it's an experience you can share with somebody else. Instead of a shiny new kitchen gadget that you'll use a few times then forget about, can you take a friend to a good meal?

STEP 3: Choose the experience over the item.

☐ If you've spent money on one fun or meaningful experience today, consider it a win.

TREAT THINGS LIKE EXPERIENCES

You make a great purchase. It's the highest-resolution, biggest-capacity, most delicious-smelling gizmo you've ever seen, and you bought it at a great price. At long last, this will be the object that brings you happiness.

One month later, your coworker shows up with a doodad that's got twice the resolution, three times the capacity, and eighteen times the olfactory delight. It cost them half as much. Also, it does their laundry.

You'd be forgiven for feeling regret.

As it happens, though, a technique can save you from comparing the stuff you bought to the stuff you didn't. Paradoxically, it relies on the fact that people are less likely to regret buying experiences than buying things (page 94).

STEP 1: Think about a purchase you once were excited about but now are comparing unfavorably to something you could have bought.

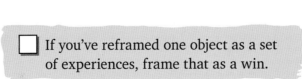

STEP 2: Consider the experiences you've had with it. What books have you read while you sat in that chair? What conversations have you had on that phone? What emotions did you feel when you watched that DVD?

☐ If you've reframed one object as a set of experiences, frame that as a win.

THINK ABOUT TUESDAY

Of course you should buy that Wi-Fi-enabled coffee cup. You can just picture yourself sitting at your desk, sipping a perfect brew, with minute-by-minute thermal tracking maintaining it at the ideal temperature.

Alas, you've just committed the sin of **focalism**—zooming in on something you hope will make you happy, without considering everything else that's going on around it. If you look at your calendar for a random day this week, you'll see that you've got back-to-back meetings at a client's office, where you won't have your SmartCup™ with you or the large, heavy charger it requires. And even quieter days end with a maddening hour-long commute. How long will your coffee-induced glow last?

Fortunately, in their book *Happy Money*, Elizabeth Dunn and Michael Norton offer a simple technique to avoid focalism: Think about a randomly chosen real-life date.

STEP 1: Identify a purchase you're considering.

. . . .

STEP 2: Think about next Tuesday, hour-by-hour. How often will you use your purchase on this specific day? When you aren't using it, how often will you think about it?

. . . .

STEP 3: Reconsider how happy you expect this purchase to make you.

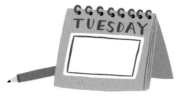

☐ If you've thought how one specific purchase will affect you on one specific day, think about today as a triumph.

BUY TIME

There is one kind of affluence that brings happiness: time affluence. The more free time you have, the happier you tend to be.

Of course, we all have the same twenty-four hours in a day. It might be more accurate to say "the more free time *you feel* you have." One way to earn that feeling is to spend more time volunteering (page 123). Paradoxically, fifteen minutes spent helping others has been shown to make people feel as if they have more free time.

Another way is simply to buy time. Consumers often focus on time-saving gadgets, and they can certainly be worthwhile. If you don't have a dishwasher or a washing machine, or another appliance that will genuinely save you time, by all means spend your disposable income to get one.

But go beyond gadgets. There are people out there who (for a fee) would love to do what you hate. Hire them, and make everybody happier.

STEP 1: Identify a way you can spend money to get more time for things you enjoy. Can you pay a neighborhood kid to mow your lawn? Or an author to come over and play with your dog for you? (You probably enjoy playing with your dog, but just in case it's an unpleasant chore, I'm available.)

STEP 2: Do a quick Think About Tuesday check (page 96) to make sure you're freeing up time on real-life days and not just imaginary ideal ones.

STEP 3: If the purchase passes Step 2, and if you can afford it, go ahead and spring for it.

☐ If you've bought time today, it's time to give yourself the win.

DO LITTLE, LOTS

Which would make you happier: $3,000 to spend on a week at the beach or $250 a month to buy a fancy meal out? Time-share salesmen might argue for the former—but psychologists advocate the latter. In a wide variety of studies, frequent small pleasures have been shown to bring more happiness than infrequent big ones.

Of all the advice in this book, this might be the most counterintuitive. Giving up lots of little pleasures to afford one big pleasure seems like the wise and mature course of action.

To understand, consider two phenomena we've already encountered. Thanks to hedonic adaptation (page 55), the boost you get from even the most decadent purchase is only temporary; making lots of little purchases lets you renew that boost again and again. And thanks to the peak-end rule (page 20), you end up with roughly the same number of memories per experience, whatever the length. Twelve distinct happy evenings will leave you with twelve distinct sets of happy memories, while that one glorious week in the sun will all blur together.

STEP 1: Think about your budget for a large discretionary purchase you've got planned.

STEP 2: Divide that budget by twelve. With that amount of money, what could you buy yourself every month? If you divided by fifty-two, what could you buy yourself every week?

STEP 3: Consider making the smaller purchases instead of the big one.

☐ If you've replaced one big, expensive pleasure with lots of smaller, cheaper pleasures, enjoy the small pleasure of victory.

SPEND ON YOUR GOALS

On page 13, I talked about cutting down on **cognitive dissonance** (the discomfort you feel when there is a difference between what you believe and what you do) and increasing your **intrinsic motivation** (the drive that comes from pursuing meaningful goals). The first step was to align your goals with your true self. Now it's time to take the next step: aligning your wallet with your goals.

STEP 1: Think about some disposable income you have.

STEP 2: Identify a goal it can help you reach. If you want to be a better swimmer, can you spend it on an hour of coaching?

STEP 3: Make the purchase, and move one step closer to your goal.

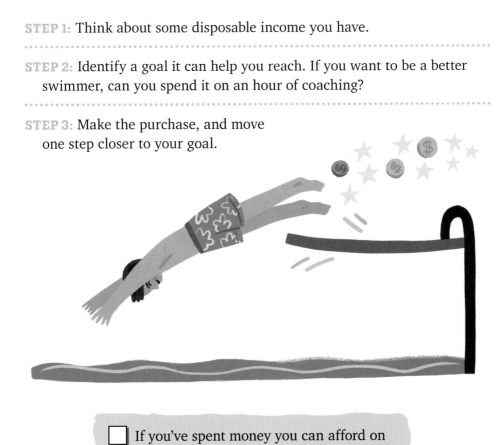

☐ If you've spent money you can afford on one of your goals, add it up as a victory.

PAY NOW, ENJOY LATER

Researchers tracked the happiness of 1,530 people, about half of whom were about to go on a trip. What they found was this:

Looking forward to vacation boosts your happiness. Actually having gone on vacation doesn't. That's right: The most happiness-boosting part of your airplane tickets is looking forward to using them.

Strange though it may sound, that's good news. Extending your vacation would cost money. But extending the looking-forward-to-your-vacation part is absolutely free.

Even outside of travel, paying for a purchase before you enjoy it gives you the added pleasure of anticipation. Buy theater tickets for later this year and you can enjoy weeks of anticipation on top of the two hours of actual performance. Or pay for a year's subscription to a brew-of-the-month club and you can look forward to new coffee beans every month. Researchers have found that people feel more happiness looking forward to a positive event than looking back on it.

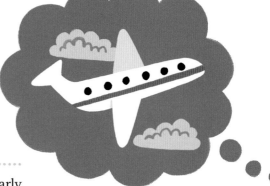

STEP 1: Find a pleasure you'd like to enjoy in the future.

STEP 2: Pay for it now.

STEP 3: Mark it on your calendar.

STEP 4: Remind yourself regularly that something good is coming.

☐ If you've prepaid for one future pleasure, or reminded yourself that one is coming, give yourself the win.

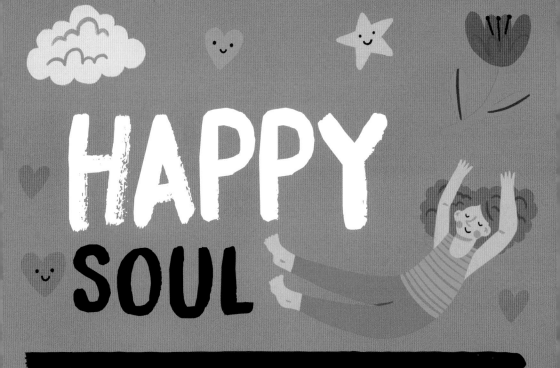

HAPPY
SOUL

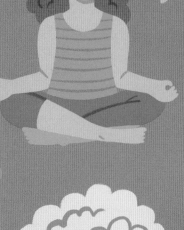

There's a certain kind of happiness that comes from deep within. Whether you believe your soul is an intangible spiritual presence or just an ordinary neurological process, this section will make it joyful.

LEARN SOME ANCIENT GREEK

For millennia, before psychologists turned their attention to happiness, philosophers were on the job. The ancient Greeks distinguished between two kinds of happiness: **hedonic happiness** comes from maximizing pleasure; **eudaemonic happiness** comes from maximizing meaning. If you're relaxing on a Caribbean beach, that's hedonic. If you're rescuing puppies, that's eudaemonic. If you're rescuing puppies on a Caribbean beach, call me. I want to be your personal assistant.

Psychologists find that people who pursue both kinds of happiness—hedonic and eudaemonic—are most likely to flourish. Philosophers probably wouldn't be surprised. Pleasure without meaning can feel empty. Meaning without pleasure can lead to burnout.

Reflecting on the difference can help you get the balance right in your own life.

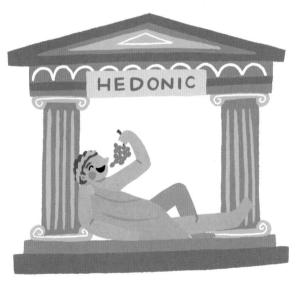

STEP 1: Think about the role of hedonic happiness in your life. What things give you pleasure? Do you do them too often, too rarely, or just the right amount?

STEP 2: Think about the role of eudaemonic happiness. What things feel meaningful and worthwhile to you? Do you do them too often, too rarely, or just the right amount?

STEP 3: Think about the trade-offs you make. Is there a time you've sacrificed meaning to get pleasure? How about vice versa? How do you feel about those trade-offs?

STEP 4: Think about times you've combined eudaemonic happiness and hedonic happiness—by having a delicious meal with people you care about, for example. Did the two kinds of happiness enhance each other? If so, do you want to combine them more often?

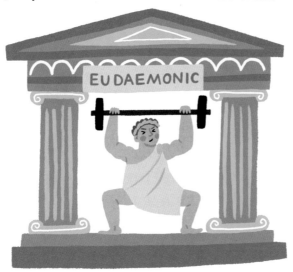

☐ If you've spent time thinking about pleasure and meaning, and how both play a role in your life, think about victory.

PUT YOURSELF IN CONTEXT

In writing this book, I've tried to be upbeat and supportive, but I've got to be honest with you: You've got some serious flaws. Don't feel bad—the same goes for Abraham Lincoln and, possibly, Dolly Parton. Flaws are part of the human condition.

This exercise combines self-compassion (page 116) with a psychological technique known as **reframing**—putting something in a new context that helps you see it more positively.

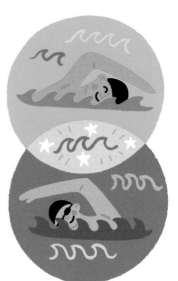

STEP 1: Think about somebody you compare yourself unfavorably with—say, that buff guy in the other lane who lapped you multiple times during your morning swim.

STEP 2: Think of a flaw that you and the other person share—for example, "We're both slower than Michael Phelps," or "We're both tired at the end of our workout."

STEP 3: Find a positive category you both belong to. In this case, it might be "People who are improving their health through exercise." Take a moment to consider that despite your mutual flaws, you and this other person have earned your right to be in that noble group.

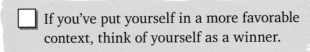

☐ If you've put yourself in a more favorable context, think of yourself as a winner.

GO AROUND THE *FEIERABEND*

Sometimes just knowing the word for something crystalizes its importance. In German, *feierabend* describes what happens from the moment you end your day's work. It's like a miniature weekend at the end of a weekday. Planning your *feierabend* means thinking about what will recharge you for the next workday. It helps you make a clean break and leave work at the office. More important, it means making sure that your personal time is personally meaningful.

STEP 1: Find a way to transition out of your workday and into your *feierabend*. Your commute might serve as a natural bridge—but if your commute is stressful and unpleasant, consider a relaxing ritual when you get home.

STEP 2: Think of your *feierabend* not just as an absence of work but as a presence of personal time. What do you want to do with the gift of free time?

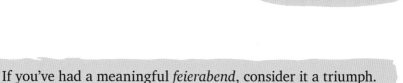

STEP 3: Live your best *feierabend*.

☐ If you've had a meaningful *feierabend*, consider it a triumph.

CONNECT WITH INSPIRATIONAL PEOPLE

In a study of the effect of inspiration on mood, scientists divided volunteers into two groups. One group watched a screen saver. The other watched a highlight reel of Michael Jordan's great dunks. Needless to say, the Jordan group felt happier afterward. Intriguingly, within the Jordan group, some were happier than others. In particular, the ones who found Michael Jordan most inspirational were the happiest.

Of course, as the researchers noted, "the conclusions are limited to the type of inspiration elicited by exposure to Michael Jordan." And so they undertook a months-long study, measuring how inspired volunteers were in their ordinary, non-Michael-Jordan-related lives. The result was the same:

Being inspired leads to gratitude and a greater purpose in life, which makes you happy.

So, whomever you look up to, spend some time contemplating them. It's a great way to dunk on sadness.

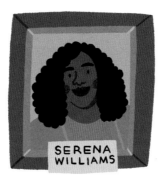

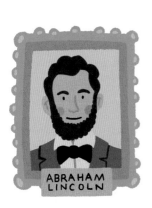

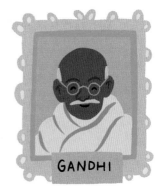

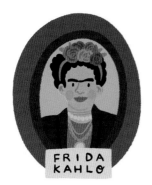

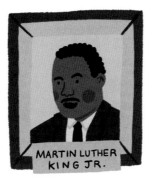

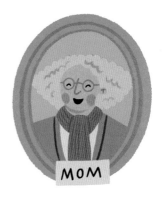

STEP 1: Think of a real-life figure, living or dead, who inspires you. It could be a world-famous figure, or it could be your mom.

STEP 2: Find a way to connect with them. Read a biography of them, for example, or listen to one of their speeches. You could even change the lock screen on your phone to be a photo of them.

STEP 3: Reflect on what this person's existence tells you about the possibilities for human achievement. What have they done that you wouldn't have thought possible? What can you do to strive, in your own imperfect way, for the ideals they represent?

STEP 4: If it's a person you know, reach out to them and tell them they inspire you (page 122).

☐ If you've thought about how one real-life figure inspires you, you're an inspirational winner.

LET YOURSELF BE MISERABLE

You might not expect this advice from a book on happiness, but . . .

Sometimes you just have to be miserable.

It's no fun to feel anger or jealousy or grief. But if that's what your circumstances make you feel, trying to convince yourself you feel chipper will make things worse. In the short term, accepting negative feelings has been shown to make them less intense, without reducing your likelihood of eventually feeling something positive. In the long term, people who habitually accept their negative feelings show more robust mental health. Indeed, years of practice in accepting sadness may be one reason that people grow happier as they age.

(Be warned, though: A series of studies have shown that accepting your life circumstances is *not* beneficial. You can accept your sadness, while still trying to change the things that make you sad.)

STEP 1: Next time you feel a negative emotion, accept that you're feeling it. You don't have to yell and break things—but you also don't have to convince yourself that you're happier than you are. If it helps, think of negative emotions as passing clouds. They're real, and they're going to cast a shadow. But as time goes by, they'll drift onward, and the sun will come out again.

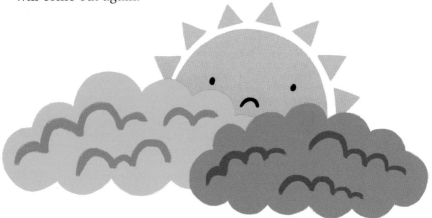

STEP 2: One way to acknowledge emotions while still lessening their pain is to translate them into words (page 27), so try to label your feelings as precisely as you can. Is it envy at somebody else's success or is it disappointment at your own failure? Or is it a complex spicy stew of both? Speaking of spicy stews, finding just the right metaphor for your feelings can help process them further. When I get anxious, I feel as if there's a volcano in my stomach and an overworked steam engine rattling in my head.

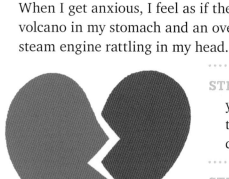

STEP 3: If you can tell somebody in your life what you're feeling (without taking it out on them!), go ahead and do so.

STEP 4: If you can take constructive action to remove the source of the emotion, do that, too. If not . . . you may just have to weather the storm.

☐ If you've accepted one negative emotion, accept that as a triumph.

IMAGINE YOU'RE WORSE OFF

If you didn't expect a book on happiness to advise that you accept negative feelings (page 108), then here's an even more surprising tip:

Sometimes you should make yourself *deliberately* sad.

The idea comes from the Stoic philosophers, who advocated imagining unpleasant things. Epictetus, for example, suggested that when you say goodbye to a friend, you consider the possibility that you will never see them again. In doing so, you confront the fear of loss and give it less power over you in the future.

Plus, although Epictetus wouldn't have used this phrase, it can help guard against hedonic adaptation. On page 55, I suggested taking a break from pleasures you enjoy regularly. But that's not suitable for every context. I wouldn't advise licking doorknobs in a hospital to take a break from being healthy, or deliberately insulting your spouse to take a break from being happily married.

Fortunately, **negative visualization** (as this technique is called) can achieve a similar result, with much lower risk of death and/or divorce.

STEP 1: Think of a positive aspect of your life—the presence of a loved one or some material comfort you're privileged to enjoy.

STEP 2: Imagine a day in your life without that good thing. How would you feel when you woke up? What changes would the absence of that good thing make to your daily happiness? What would you do to try to get back what you lost?

STEP 3: Back in the real world, feel a new appreciation for your good fortune.

> ☐ If you've used negative visualization to appreciate one good thing, appreciate the victory.

ACT PLAYFUL, GET JOYFUL

Playfulness has been good for our species, helping us work together and stumble across vital discoveries. And it turns out to be equally good for us as individuals. Playful people display higher levels of happiness and more constructive uses of humor.

I'm not talking about some obsessive competition where you grind out a win or die. Play ought to be . . . well, playful. Some psychologists define playfulness as the ability to make everyday situations interesting or entertaining. Kicking over a chessboard when you lose won't make you happy. Acting out *Romeo and Juliet* with your clothes as you do the laundry will. (And if your kids give you funny looks, tell them it's for their own good. Kids with playful parents grow up to have more positive outlooks in life.)

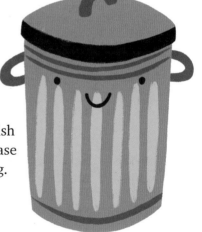

STEP 1: Think about something you don't normally approach playfully, like taking out the trash, or getting your kids to do their homework.

STEP 2: Make it playful. Give your trash can a name. Promise your kids that if they finish their homework, you'll insert the silly phrase of their choice into the book you're writing. (Incidentally, I'm a big poo-poo head, and my nose is made of cheese.)

☐ If you've brought a sense of play to one new activity, playfully accept the victory.

MEDITATE

Relative to the thousands of years that humanity has practiced meditation, scientists have only begun studying it recently. Current evidence suggests it reduces stress, boosts happiness, makes pain less unpleasant, improves self-control, and has a host of other physical and mental benefits. It's possible that meditation does even more than we currently think.

But it's also possible that it does *less*, or that its benefits change depending on the kind of meditation we're doing.

Admittedly, something like that is true for every entry in this book. Scientists are constantly rethinking old beliefs in light of new evidence, and that's especially true when we're dealing with the hard-to-measure world of human emotions. I'm only expressing more skepticism about meditation than my other tips because meditation has received more hype than, say, napping or eating fruit.

I hope you find that meditation adds a lot to your life. It certainly has to mine! I just don't want you to be disappointed if it doesn't give you superpowers, or to feel inferior if you're the only person at a dinner party who hasn't tried it yet.

If you'd like guidance from an experienced meditation teacher, sign up for a local meditation class or download a meditation app to your phone. If you'd like to give it a go on your own, try the simple exercise below.

STEP 1: Sit comfortably in a quiet place. If this is your first time meditating, set a timer for a short and manageable time. Even a minute is fine—everybody has to start somewhere!

STEP 2: Close your eyes, and focus on your breath. Notice how your chest rises and falls. If your mind wanders, that's natural. Just calmly and without any judgment bring your attention back to your breath.

STEP 3: Let your attention flow to your feet. Notice, without judgment, what sensations they currently feel. Let your attention flow upward until you reach the top of your head.

STEP 4: Repeat Step 2, Step 3, or both until your meditation period has ended.

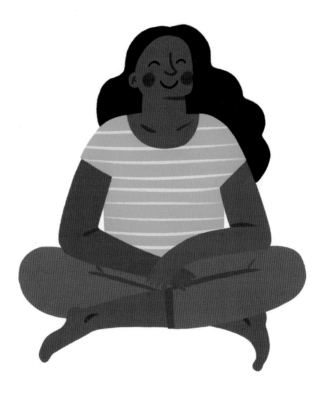

☐ If you meditated, meditate on your win.

MAKE PROCRASTINATION WORK FOR YOU

We all do things we know we shouldn't. Maybe it's texting a particularly toxic ex, or it's eating one M&M too many. Or, for the black widow spiders among you, maybe it's eating one ex too many. Even as we're doing these things, we know they'll end in misery, or at the very least regret.

Fortunately, a psychological technique can help us resist the lure of those delicious, crunchy exes. It's called **unspecific postponement.** Instead of telling yourself you mustn't give in to temptation, you tell yourself you'll do it some other time.

Unspecific postponement has been shown to be effective at resisting short-term temptation. Over the long term, it can actually reduce your desire for whatever it is you're resisting. One possible reason? By putting off doing it, you signal to yourself that you don't really value it.

STEP 1: Next time you feel tempted to do something that you know will make you unhappy, don't try to stop yourself from doing it ever. Just tell yourself you'll do it some other time.

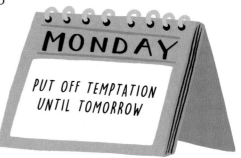

STEP 2: If the temptation recurs, tell yourself the same thing.

☐ If you've put off one temptation to an unspecified time, don't put off taking the win.

BE COMPASSIONATE TOWARD ALL

According to the Dalai Lama, "Compassion has two functions: It causes our brain to function better, and it brings inner strength. These, then, are the causes of happiness." Science agrees: Compassion has been found to correlate with **eudaemonia**, or the happiness of personal meaning (page 102).

STEP 1: Think about any other living being in the world. If you want to really challenge your compassion skills, make it somebody you don't like.

STEP 2: Think of a flaw they have or a misfortune they've suffered. Reflect on how their flaw or suffering gives them something in common with you.

STEP 3: Putting aside your thoughts of yourself, empathize with their suffering and feel the desire to help them.

STEP 4: It may not be practical to help that particular person at this particular moment. But if you feel inspired to act, you have plenty of options—see page 123.

> ☐ If you've felt compassion for another living being, you are a compassionate winner.

BE COMPASSIONATE TO YOURSELF, TOO

It's easier to be compassionate toward others than to ourselves. But self-compassion is a deeply valuable tool. Recent studies suggest it has the positive psychological effect of self-esteem, but without the risk of narcissism and arrogance that high self-esteem can bring.

This exercise comes from Dr. Kristin Neff, a psychology professor and expert in self-compassion.

STEP 1: Get out a piece of paper and a pen, or sit down at your computer, phone, or tablet.

STEP 2: Write down the kinds of things you would typically say to a friend who is feeling bad about themself. Write down not just the words but anything you know about your own body language—the tone of voice you would use, for example, or how you might stand.

STEP 3: Now write down the kinds of things you say and do to *yourself* when you're feeling bad about yourself.

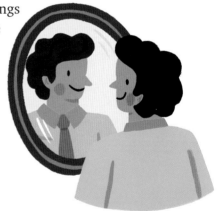

STEP 4: Compare the two. Do you treat yourself with less compassion?

STEP 5: Finally, write down how you think you might feel if you treated yourself with the same kindness and compassion you show your friends.

☐ If you've done a self-compassion exercise, or put self-compassion into real-life practice, give yourself the win . . . In fact, you know what? Give yourself the win no matter what.

CHOOSE A HAPPY PLACE

Suddenly, the building catches fire. Burning timbers plummet all around you, and one of your friends is feeling his pulse pound as the full enormity of the situation hits him. A different friend is thinking about that time she went sailing with her grandpa. Which one is better equipped to help you all escape?

If you said the sailor, you're right.

In one study, psychologists stimulated the stress response of volunteers by having them plunge their hands into icy water. Then they asked half the group to recall a happy memory and the other half to think about something neutral. When they measured levels of the stress hormone cortisol, they found that the happy reminiscers had significantly less than the neutral group, not to mention less negative emotion overall.

Whether you're in a burning building or just facing a stressful commute, staying calm under pressure can help you navigate to a happy ending. And you can lay the groundwork for it right now.

STEP 1: Think about a happy memory you'd like to return to—a time you cuddled with your dog or a relaxing family trip. The more sensory details you can summon, the better.

STEP 2: Make a mental note that the next time you feel stressed, you should summon up that memory. You can even practice in advance by plunging your hands into ice water and then calming yourself with reminiscences.

STEP 3: Next time you feel stressed, take a moment to immerse yourself in the memory you've chosen. It will calm you down enough to think rationally about your situation and take the steps to improve it.

☐ If you've returned to a happy memory in times of stress, or even just chosen a memory you'll return to, look back on this as a triumph.

CHANGE IT UP

You're trying to decide whether to make some change in your life. Should you start a new diet? Break up with your boyfriend? Quit your job?

Sometimes you lean one way or the other . . . but sometimes it's essentially a coin toss.

In those cases, you should consider an experiment by *Freakonomics* author Steven D. Levitt. He set up a website for people torn about life decisions. It provided them with a virtual coin toss to tell them which way to go. In exchange, they had to check back two months later, and again six months later, and report whether the change had made them happier.

Twenty thousand people participated. And by a significant margin, the people who reported the greatest increase in happiness were those who made a change.

Or, at least, made a *big* change. Getting a new hairstyle didn't seem to enhance anybody's long-term happiness. Breaking up with a bad partner, starting a new business, or moving did.

Levitt's conclusion? Most people have a bias against change, which makes them hesitant about changing their life in a way that will ultimately make them happier.

STEP 1: Think about a change you're tempted to make, but you really could go either way on.

STEP 2: Consider all the rational and emotional reasons, pro and con, to see if you can come to a reasoned conclusion. Also do a gut check to see if you have a strong feeling about which direction you should go in.

STEP 3: If, after all that, you still can't decide . . . make the change.

> ☐ If you've made one change you've been agonizing over, conclude that it's a victory.

GO WEST, YOUNG MAN. THEN EAST. THEN TRY NORTH.

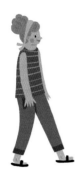
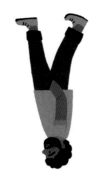

Researchers tracked the locations of 132 volunteers for more than three months via their phones and periodically sent them text messages to check in on their mood. The happiest people were those who had visited a variety of places during the day and had spent about the same amount of time in each of them.

Researchers also brought about half the volunteers into the lab and gave them MRI scans, trying to learn more about the neural mechanism at work. They found an association between the hippocampus (which processes novel experiences) and the striatum (an important part of the brain's reward mechanism).

STEP 1: If you can, include a variety of environments in your day, giving yourself equal chance to experience them.

STEP 2: If that's not possible, figure out how to inject at least a little bit of novelty into your life. Can you take a different route to work? Swap seats every fifteen minutes at dinner?

☐ If you've explored multiple environments by making even a small change to your normal routine today, give yourself the win.

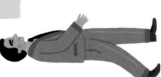

TURN OFF—*BUZZ!*
SORRY, TURN OFF YOUR—*BING!*

That parade of electronic notifications doesn't just shatter your attention. Studies show that it shatters your happiness, too. That's because distractions interfere with mindfulness: You can't enjoy the moment if your phone is desperately trying to remind you of four undone tasks, eighteen future events, and a hundred unpleasant things happening somewhere in the world.

Fortunately, most electronics give you a bunch of options for managing notifications. See the sidebar if you're not familiar with the vocabulary. Then dive in, and tell your phone to shut up and mind its own business.

The Language of Distraction

- A *badge* is a little symbol that pops up on top of an app.

- A *notification center* is a place where you can review notifications that have come in. It's usually something you can choose to go to when you're ready, rather than be interrupted whenever the notifications come in.

- A *pop-up window* is a little box that pops up on your screen, possibly covering up that photo you took of a beautiful rose with an ominous email from your accountant.

STEP 1: Go to the notifications settings on your phone. Turn every single one off.

STEP 2: Now go through them again, and for each one, follow the flow chart.

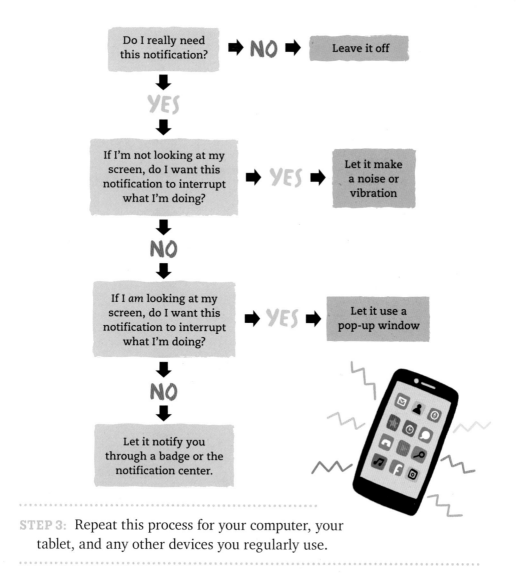

Do I really need this notification? ➡ **NO** ➡ Leave it off

YES

If I'm not looking at my screen, do I want this notification to interrupt what I'm doing? ➡ **YES** ➡ Let it make a noise or vibration

NO

If I *am* looking at my screen, do I want this notification to interrupt what I'm doing? ➡ **YES** ➡ Let it use a pop-up window

NO

Let it notify you through a badge or the notification center.

STEP 3: Repeat this process for your computer, your tablet, and any other devices you regularly use.

STEP 4: Whenever you install a new app, get in the habit of clicking "No" when it asks if it can notify you.

☐ If you've turned off at least one notification, notify yourself of your win.

GIVE THANKS

Happy people don't necessarily have more good things—they just appreciate the good things they have. Based on numerous studies, deliberately exercising your gratitude muscles can bring an immediate happiness boost while developing a skill that will increase your long-term life satisfaction.

STEP 1: Start a gratitude journal. Every day, write down one thing from the past twenty-four hours that you're grateful for.

STEP 2: Contact somebody you have a current relationship with, and tell them why you're grateful for them.

STEP 3: For an advanced gratitude boost, think about somebody from your past whom you never sufficiently thanked for a good deed. Write a letter thanking them, and make sure they get it.

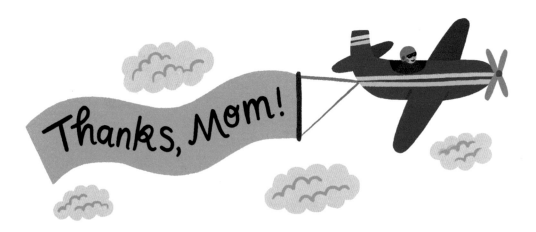

☐ If you've done one gratitude exercise today, be grateful for the victory.

HELP!

Volunteering increases life expectancy, reduces the risk of depression, and increases feelings of energy and joy. If volunteering were a drug, it would be dangerously addictive, but if people volunteered at rehab centers, they'd only make the problem worse.

Interestingly, the mental benefits of volunteering vary with age. For folks over sixty-five, it has a major effect. Between forty and sixty-five, it has *some* effect. Under forty, volunteering is still admirable—but it doesn't improve your overall life satisfaction. Psychologists are still investigating why. It may be that the more established you feel in your career, the freer you are to seek meaning in unpaid work.

STEP 1: Identify a nonprofit organization in your area with a mission you believe in.

STEP 2: Find out how you can volunteer to help them out. If you can't make it there in person, you might be able to volunteer remotely. When I found myself thousands of miles away from my home state during an important election, I volunteered for a get-out-the-vote group, contacting voters from the comfort of my own computer. It was immensely satisfying.

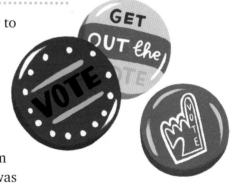

STEP 3: Sign up, show up, and cheer up.

☐ If you've volunteered for a good cause, volunteer to accept your winner's trophy.

SAY NO

Warren Buffett once said, "The difference between successful people and *very* successful people is that very successful people say 'no' to almost everything."

Advice on how to get rich doesn't usually overlap with advice on how to be happy, but this is a rare exception. Overcommitment correlates with increased stress and cynicism, and decreased efficiency. Why make yourself less happy in order to make yourself less successful?

I knew a woman who stuck a list labeled "Ways to Say No" on the wall next to her phone. She was a bestselling author, and she didn't need help remembering the words *no*, *thank*, and *you*. She just needed to remember that she was allowed to use them.

Ways to Say No

- That won't be possible.
- I appreciate the offer, but it's not right for me.
- I've had to cut back on my commitments lately.
- No, thank you.
- I'm afraid I can't do that. Thank you for thinking of me, though.
- I'm flattered, but I'm not really qualified to be Queen of England.

STEP 1: Next time somebody asks you to do something, resist the urge to immediately say yes. If you need a reminder, post a list of Ways to Say No next to your landline or stick it to the back of your cell phone.

STEP 2: Pause to think about it. Are you saying yes because you really, truly want to do whatever is being asked of you? Or do you feel pressure from the other person or your own sense of guilt? Sometimes you have to say yes because it's truly your moral duty to help. But otherwise . . . as the saying goes, "If it's not a *Hell yes!* it's a *No*.

STEP 3: Unless you want to say *Hell yes!*, say *No*.

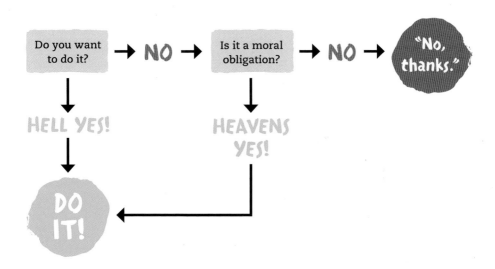

If you've said *No* to one thing that was neither a pleasure nor a genuine moral duty, say *Yes!* to giving yourself credit.

FEEL AWE-SOME

Given that awe is the appreciation of the vast and the unknowable, you wouldn't think it amenable to scientific study. In fact, psychologists have figured out how to induce it and then to track its consequences—a pretty awe-inspiring achievement in itself.

What they found is that awe inspires profound feelings of humility (a crucial ingredient in happy relationships) and happiness.

STEP 1: Put yourself in a position to experience awe. Visit a cathedral or a cathedral-size tree, or check out a book on the Grand Canyon, or just search "size of the universe" on your favorite video website and watch the results.

STEP 2: Let yourself experience not just awe but also the humility and calm that follows.

STEP 3: After letting yourself dwell on the experience for a little while, make a mental note of it. Remembering an experience of awe has been shown to have similar benefits to experiencing it.

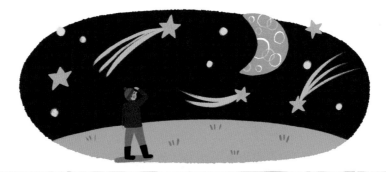

☐ If you've given yourself an experience of awe and humility today, give yourself a galaxy-size check mark.

FIGHT NIGEL

Having an inner critic isn't a bad thing. People who never second-guess themselves are more likely to jump out of an airplane without confirming they've got a parachute. (Or so I'm guessing. Surprisingly few scientific studies involve shoving people out of planes.)

But when your inner critic gets too loud and vociferous, it can drown out your joy in life. Fortunately, there's a way to listen to your inner critic without taking it too seriously. It comes from Julia Cameron, and it's a variation on the principle of **cognitive defusion** (page 30). Cameron has written more than forty books, including *The Artist's Way*, so her relationship with her inner critic seems to be working pretty well.

STEP 1: Assign your inner critic a name. Cameron calls hers "Nigel."

STEP 2: Think about what kind of person would say the things your inner critic tends to say. Use that information to develop a personality for your critic. Are they a cranky octogenarian? A spoiled toddler?

STEP 3: The next time a voice in your head criticizes your choices, picture it coming from the person you've identified. Tell them you'll take their advice under consideration, then dismiss them.

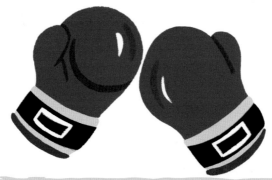

☐ If you've dismissed your inner critic by name, give yourself the win.

DANCE YOUR TROUBLES AWAY

Music makes you happy—but you have to put a little work into it. In a survey of one thousand people, those who interacted with music by dancing or going to live concerts were happier with their lives than people who just listened to music (or, heaven forbid, led musicless lives).

Researchers think dancing is effective because it combines emotional self-expression with physical activity, while going to concerts is an inherently social experience.

STEP 1: Put on a favorite song.

STEP 2: Dance to it.

STEP 3: If a band you like is performing in your area, get tickets and go. (Long-term happiness tip: Take earplugs, and use them if the music is loud enough to drown out a normal speaking voice. The longer you've got working eardrums, the longer they can bring you joy.)

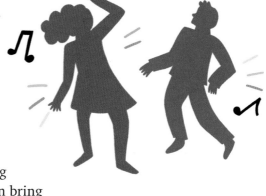

☐ If you've danced to a song or attended a concert, dance to victory.

LAUGH IT UP

People with good senses of humor are happier in just about every measure. They're less likely to suffer from depression, they recover faster from illness, and they have higher life satisfaction.

In the long term, you can do plenty of things to develop your sense of humor. Sign up for an improv comedy class, or start performing at open-mic nights. For that matter, just have kids.

But in the short term, there's a simple exercise you can do today. It's one of the rare humor exercises that's been tested in a double-blind study.

STEP 1: Think of three funny things you saw today. Write them down, in as much detail as you can. Don't worry about making your writing funny, or even grammatical. You're not submitting this to *The New Yorker*. You're just exercising your ability to spot funny stuff.

STEP 2: If you can't think of three funny things, seek them out. Look up your favorite comedian on Twitter, search for "funny" on a video website, or watch a scene from your favorite comedy.

STEP 3: Tomorrow, keep an eye out for humor as you go about your day.

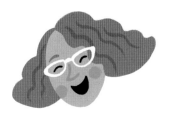  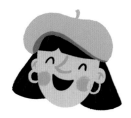

☐ If you can think of three funny things you've seen today, laugh all the way to the winner's podium.

CELEBRATE THE SEASONS

Earlier, I mentioned that taking a break from a pleasure can help get you off the hedonic treadmill (page 55). For the same effect with less willpower, let the calendar do the work for you. It's no challenge to give up drinking hot chocolate when it's 100 degrees Fahrenheit outside. Plus, in a year salted with seasonal pleasures, you'll always have something to look forward to.

I'd particularly encourage you to seek out delights associated with the season you like the least. Reframing is a psychologically healthy way to deal with unpleasant situations, and if you can reframe February from "The month I freeze my tush off" to "The month of the Great Neighborhood Snowball Battle," you're on your way to happiness.

And remember: There are more seasons than summer, autumn, winter, and spring. On my calendar, I've marked out strawberry and plum seasons as well. As I write this, it's a cold and dark January day, but looking forward to the sweet taste of the future is bringing me cheer. Some seasons (like Olympic season) come less than once a year, giving you even longer to enjoy the anticipation.

STEP 1: Enjoy what's unique to the current season.

STEP 2: Get out your calendar, and plan some celebrations for the rest of the year. That way, you can enjoy the anticipation as well as the practice.

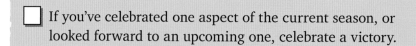

☐ If you've celebrated one aspect of the current season, or looked forward to an upcoming one, celebrate a victory.

Things to Look Forward to All Year

Summer
- The smell of sunscreen
- Trips to the beach
- Late sunsets
- Baseball

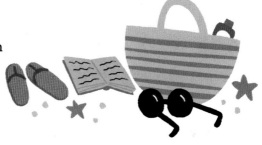

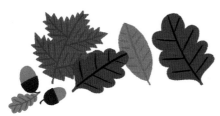

Autumn
- The smell of leaves
- Sleeping late as the days shorten
- All the rituals of a new school year
- Football season

Winter
- Snowball fights
- Hot chocolate
- Ice-skating
- Hearing Christmas carols everywhere you go
- Christmas being over, and not having to hear Christmas carols for an entire year

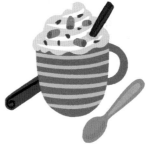

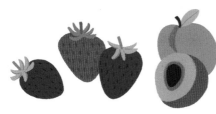

Spring
- Strawberries and apricots
- Baseball spring training
- Flowers blooming
- Packing away winter clothing

MAKE IT A HABIT

Throughout the book, I've labeled activities that I think would make great habits. But what *is* a habit, exactly?

A habit is something you do often enough to reach a state of **automaticity**—that is, to do it without thinking. There's no magic number of repetitions to reach automaticity. It varies from person to person and habit to habit. One study showed it can take as few as 18 days or as many as 254, with an average time of 66 days.

So what makes a habit habitual? Psychologists say it's the cycle of *trigger, action,* and *reward.*

STEP 1: Identify a habit you want to acquire. Let's say it's going for a run through your local park.

STEP 2: Choose a trigger for the habit. Ideally, this will be some concrete thing you already do regularly. If you feed your cat every morning, try putting your running shoes next to her dish, allowing you to stack a new habit on top of an old one. You can even link your new habit to an existing *bad* habit, by deciding you won't check Twitter until you've gone for a run. This is called **temptation bundling**.

STEP 3: Think about a reward your new habit will lead to. This might be an immediate benefit (like an endorphin rush) or a long-term goal (like having more energy as you get more fit).

STEP 4: Do your desired action as soon as the trigger occurs.

STEP 5: Enjoy the reward (if it's something immediate) or the anticipation of it (if it's more long term).

STEP 6: For an extra motivation boost, consider tracking your habit. Even the small gesture of making a check mark can be its own reward.

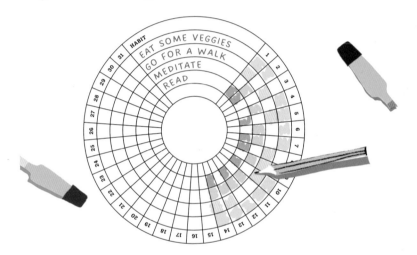

Turn the tips from this book into daily, weekly, monthly, and lifelong habits with the helpful habit trackers inside this jacket! Copy or trace these trackers, then customize them to track habits, increase mindfulness, and help reach your goals!

☐ If you've started one happy habit (or kept a happy habit streak going), you've made a habit out of victory.

SEEK PROFESSIONAL HELP: A BONUS TIP

I believe the tips in this book will help you live a happier life. But I also believe that there are limits to what a book can do. Sometimes you need a real flesh-and-blood human who understands what you're going through and can help you get through it.

If you got run over, you wouldn't hesitate to seek professional help for your body. Sometimes life is a Zamboni aimed right at your soul. There are people whose job is to help peel you off the ice. Reach out to them.

Signs You Might Benefit from Therapy

- You feel overwhelmingly helpless for an extended period.
- Things don't get better no matter what you try.
- You can't do your everyday tasks at work or home.
- You are constantly worried or anxious.
- You're navigating a particularly challenging life event.
- You have a chronic physical illness that's negatively affecting your emotional life.
- You're doing something that's harming you or the people around you.
- You just need a nonjudgmental ear to listen while you talk.

STEP 1: Reflect on whether any of the signs in the sidebar apply to you.

STEP 2: If so, find a mental health care professional. Some ways to do that:

- Get a recommendation from a friend or family member, or a referral from your doctor.

- If your unhappiness is related to a specific challenge you're facing, ask for a referral from a related profession. A divorce attorney might know somebody who can help you cope with divorce, and a physical therapist might know somebody who can help you with the mental effects of injury.

- Get a referral through your insurance plan.

- Get in touch with your local community health center, or the psychology department of a local university.

- Contact your local psychological association. You can find a list of them here: apa.org/about/apa/organizations/associations

- Use the American Psychological Association's online locator: locator.apa.org

STEP 3: Book an appointment.

STEP 4: Show up for it.

STEP 5: After the appointment, decide if you would like to see that therapist again. If not, that's okay—think of this as a first date. Just as you wouldn't stop dating if you had one bad evening, don't stop seeking a psychotherapist after one bad session. Keep trying until you find a therapist you connect with. It will be worth it.

☐ If you've had an appointment with a mental health care professional—or even booked one—give yourself the win.

Acknowledgments

I'm happy to have a lot of wonderful people helping me with this book.

In 2019, my agent, Joan Paquette, recognized that I'd click with the brilliant and passionate staff of Odd Dot and suggested I stop by their offices and meet them. That meeting has led to three books so far. Thank you, Joan, for that and for your ongoing insight, support, and cheerleading.

And speaking of Odd Dot's brilliant and passionate staff, thank you to Daniel Nayeri, Nathalie Le Du, Tim Hall, Christina Quintero, Caitlyn Hunter, Kate Avino, Jen Healey, Barbara Cho, Kathy Wielgosz, and Tracy Koontz. Special thanks to my editor, Justin Krasner, for bringing me on to this project and pushing me to make it the best it could be.

Thank you to Matthew D. Della Porta, PhD, cofounder of Lean Positive, LLC, who reviewed this manuscript and helped me understand the science. If I got things wrong despite his patience and care, that is entirely my fault.

Above all, thank you to my wife, Lauren, and my children, Erin and Joe, for their tolerance and compassion during the many weekends and evenings I disappeared into my office to work on this book. The three of you make me happier now, and always.

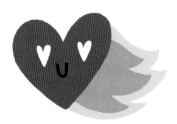